Decision-Making,
Personhood
and Dementia

of related interest

Ethical Issues in Dementia Care
Making Difficult Decisions
Julian C. Hughes and Clive Baldwin
ISBN 978 1 84310 357 8
Bradford Dementia Group Good Practice Guides

Person-Centred Counselling for People with Dementia
Making Sense of Self
Danuta Lipinska
Foreword by Brian Thorne
ISBN 978 1 84310 978 5

Understanding Care Homes
A Research and Development Perspective
Edited by Katherine Froggatt, Sue Davies and Julienne Meyer
ISBN 978 1 84310 553 4

Early Psychosocial Interventions in Dementia
Evidence-Based Practice
Edited by Esme Moniz-Cook and Jill Manthorpe
ISBN 978 1 84310 683 8

Involving Families in Care Homes
A Relationship-Centred Approach to Dementia Care
Bob Woods, John Keady and Diane Seddon
ISBN 978 1 84310 229 8
Bradford Dementia Group Good Practice Guides

Remembering Yesterday, Caring Today
Reminiscence in Dementia Care: A Guide to Good Practice
Pam Schweitzer and Errollyn Bruce
Foreword by Faith Gibson
ISBN 978 1 84310 649 4
Bradford Dementia Group Good Practice Guides

Decision-Making, Personhood and Dementia

Exploring the Interface

Edited by Deborah O'Connor
and Barbara Purves

Jessica Kingsley Publishers
London and Philadelphia

First published in 2009
by Jessica Kingsley Publishers
116 Pentonville Road
London N1 9JB, UK
and
400 Market Street, Suite 400
Philadelphia, PA 19106, USA

www.jkp.com

Library of Congress Cataloging in Publication Data

Decision-making, personhood and dementia : exploring the interface / edited by Deborah O'Connor and Barbara Purves.
p. cm.
ISBN 978-1-84310-585-5 (pb : alk. paper) 1. Dementia. 2. Decision-making. I. O'Connor, Deborah. II. Purves, Barbara.
RC521.D43 2009
616.8'3--dc22
2008048908

British Library Cataloguing in Publication Data
A CIP catalogue record for this book is available from the British Library

ISBN 978 1 84310 585 5

Printed and bound in Great Britain by
Athenaeum Press, Gateshead, Tyne and Wear

Contents

Acknowledgements

We wish to acknowledge with gratitude three funding agencies which were pivotal to the completion of this project. First, we would like to acknowledge the infrastructure support that we receive through the Michael Smith Foundation for Health Research (MSFHR). This funding has been critical for establishing the Centre for Research on Personhood in Dementia (CRPD), which brings together researchers from across disciplines to explore the personal, interpersonal, and social influences on the dementia experience in order to find ways to improve quality of life for persons with dementia and their families. Discussions within the CRPD provided the foundation for initiating this project.

Second, grants through the Social Sciences and Humanities Research Council (SSHRC) and the Canadian Institutes on Health Research (Institute on Aging) provided the funding which enabled us to bring together a small group of interdisciplinary, international researchers to talk and think about issues related to personhood, dementia, and decision-making for two days in May 2007. This workshop provided the impetus for this book, and we are indeed grateful for the funding we received to host the initial workshop.

We are also truly grateful for the support of staff and students at the CRPD in preparing this volume. We particularly wish to thank Vicky Duffield, Marcus Greatheart, Sally Clark, and Jasmyne Rockwell for their enthusiastic and skilled assistance.

Finally, the quality of an edited volume is ultimately dependent on the commitment of its contributors. We are indebted to all those who contributed chapters to this volume, for their willingness to share their ideas and their patience throughout this process.

Introduction

CHAPTER 1

Decision-Making, Personhood and Dementia
Mapping the Terrain

DEBORAH O'CONNOR AND BARBARA PURVES

INTRODUCTION: DEMENTIA AND DECISION-MAKING

Dementia is a devastating disorder which may dramatically interfere with health, well-being and quality of life of both the person with the diagnosis and his or her family. Historically, it has been viewed largely as a biomedical phenomenon with a trajectory of irrevocable decline related to neurodegenerative changes. Deteriorating memory, insight, judgement and ability to communicate are included as symptoms of this disorder. Using this lens, it is assumed that, over time, the person with dementia will become progressively more dependent upon others for all aspects of his or her care.

Superimposed into any discussions of dementia are issues associated with decision-making. Commonly, these are translated into deliberations about 'capacity' or 'competence' (or conversely, incapacity and incompetence). These two terms, capacity and competence, are generally seen as two related but distinct concepts typically associated with *formal* assessments of decision-making. A common method for distinguishing between the two is that capacity denotes a clinical status that is determined by a healthcare professional, while competence refers to a legal status as judged by a legal professional (see for example Marson and Briggs 2001; Shulman, Cohen and Hull 2005, p.26). Royall (2002) extends this distinction in a somewhat different way, noting that 'capacity can be thought of as a functional ability intrinsic to the individual whereas competency is a social status conveyed upon them' (p.1885). His definition moves beyond the health/legal divide and begins to capture the shift that is currently underway from more global notions of competence to more specific assessments of capacity; this will be the usage we will draw on. Using this definition, capacity can be operationalized as the ability to perform a certain task or make a specific decision (see for example Kluge 2005; Moye and Marson 2007). Generally the decisions where capacity is under consideration centre on formal issues such as driving, financial management, ability to live independently, testamentary capacity and ability to give informed consent or legal directives.

Given the emergence of individualism and the hypercognitive society (Post 2000), it is not surprising that discussions related to decision-making have typically centred around these concepts of capacity and competence, with a particular focus on assessing to determine if present or not. As Moye and Marson (2007) note, the 'field of capacity assessments is dominated by a funda-mental tension between two core ethical principles: autonomy (self-determina-tion) and protection (beneficence)' (p.P3). Conventionally, an assessment of capacity has provided the framework for resolving this tension – although whether it is a good framework is subject to considerable debate. (See 'Conclu-sion', this volume). Thus, when considering the predicament of someone with dementia, discussions about decision-making have a tendency quickly to resort to a focus on whether or not that person is capable of making a particular decision or taking a particular action. This determination generally draws on at least one of four common standards for evaluating: evidencing a choice, under-standing relevant information, appreciating the significance of that informa-tion for one's own situation and demonstrating the ability to reason. Once deemed incapable, rights to self-determination typically take a backseat to protection.

There are two points to be made here. First, discussions about decision-making related to dementia have most frequently revolved around decision-making within more formal realms of life. It is recognized that this captures only a very small part of the picture since, in practice, many situations of diminished capacity are handled informally, often by the family. Second, although decision-making is a more inclusive term – which goes beyond a simple discussion of capacity, or even the broader notion of competence, to allow for a more comprehensive appraisal of both abilities and process – to date, this discussion has typically been restricted to examining issues related to the determination of capacity.

This discussion has disadvantaged people with dementia. Too frequently, an implicit assumption underpinning interactions with members of this group is that they are indeed 'incapable'. For example, the voices of persons with dementia have historically been unheard in research because there have been assumptions, first, that they cannot give informed consent and, second, that they have so little insight into their own experiences that they would not be able to contribute anyway. This has not been intentional exclusion; rather the presence of the dementia diagnosis was tacitly understood to mean that active participation in decision-making was no longer possible. Research is now emerging that demonstrates the inaccuracy of this assumption (see for example Bond *et al.* 2002; Clare *et al.* 2008; Woods and Pratt 2005). Hence, with a growing focus on recognizing people with dementia as citizens (see Bartlett and O'Connor 2007), this exclusion is being challenged and new policies and legislations are being developed expressly to counter assumptions about incapability. For example, in Canada, several provinces have either introduced, or are introducing, new substitute decision-making legislation – all begin by reiterating the guiding principle that competence is presumed, and some explicitly shift the focus to an assessment of incapability rather than capability. Similarly, in England, the Mental Capacity Act 2005 is seen as 'enshrining a legal right to autonomy' for people with dementia even when they lack capacity, thus advancing civil and social rights through an emphasis on protecting liberty, promoting self-determination and providing social rights to facilitate autonomy (Boyle 2008).

Understanding decision-making in people with dementia is targeted as a research and practice priority (Moye and Marson 2007). In particular, the need to develop a more robust theory of decision-making that extends beyond the parameters of assessing cognition has been targeted (Kluge 2005; see also Moye *et al.* 2007).

INTEGRATING PERSONHOOD: TOWARD A SOCIAL MODEL OF CARE

Despite its importance, however, understanding of issues related to decision-making in dementia remains murky at best. In fact, rather than becoming clearer, the water is further muddied as the biomedical lens is increasingly challenged with respect to its ability to offer a broad enough vision of the dementia experience. Newer perspectives recognize that the performance, behaviour and quality of life of persons with dementia are determined not only by neuropathology but also by their personal histories, their interactions with others and by how they are perceived within their social contexts. Growing evidence indicates that at least some of the negative consequences associated with dementia may be mitigated or delayed by an approach to care that respects and supports each individual's personhood and that facilitates its transformation and development throughout the disease.

Tom Kitwood was one of the first to draw attention to personhood in the context of dementia care. As a social psychologist, he identified how social interactions in the care environment could profoundly affect persons with dementia, and argued for a model of care that would recognize and support personhood throughout the course of the disease. He defined personhood as 'the standing or status that is bestowed upon one human being, by others, in the context of relationship and social being' (Kitwood 1997, p.8). With this shift to a focus on personhood, the retention of personal and social identities beyond that of dementia patient emerges as a critical issue in dementia care. This approach to care, referenced in a variety of ways, including person-centred care, social interactionist approach and, most recently, relational care, is based on concepts of interdependence and relationship (see for example Cheston and Bender 1999; Harding and Palfrey 1997; Kitwood 1997; Nolan *et al.* 2003).

The idea that personhood is socially constructed and maintained seems intuitive. However, as Harrison (1993) points out, this understanding actually challenges traditional philosophically based views (e.g. Buchanan and Brock 1989) that link autonomy with personhood as the basis of moral agency. In this view, personhood requires high-level cognitive abilities, such as consciousness, rationality, intentionality, memory, reciprocity and the ability to communicate. Because dementia is associated with a progressive decline in these cognitive functions, the disease has historically been assumed to strip the individual of his or her personhood status, leading to a 'loss of self' (Cohen and Eisdorfer 1986). By contrast, Kitwood's notion of personhood disentangles personhood from autonomy and cognitive function; hence, his broader conceptualization can apply to persons even with severely compromised cognitive functions. Within the past decade, this new way of thinking about dementia has triggered exciting research focused on trying to better understand how personhood – or sense of one's self as a unique person with a distinct entity – is maligned, maintained and/or fostered during the dementia experience, since this is seen as critical to quality of life and functioning.

While some may argue that such differences in conceptualizations of personhood simply reflect differences within the project of philosophy versus that of social psychology, it is nonetheless the case that, as Post points out, 'ideas have consequences' (2000, p.248). In other words, the implications of drawing on broader, less cognitively based conceptualizations of personhood, or selfhood, to create new understandings of decision-making in dementia, are huge. In particular, this lens leads to a more iterative understanding of capacity that is fluid, complex and relational. It also introduces the notion that decisional ability may not be the only, or even the most important, element influencing the decision-making process, particularly at the informal level.

PERSONHOOD, DEMENTIA AND DECISION-MAKING: EXPLORING THE INTERFACE

To date, the interface between this social/relational approach to personhood and decision-making for and by persons with dementia has remained relatively unexplored. Rarely has the literature concerning a social constructionist or personhood-centred approach to dementia care intersected with the health and legal literature around decision-making. Rather, as already noted, research in the area of decision-making has placed considerable effort on trying to determine when a person is no longer capable of making particular decisions and/or is globally incompetent. With very few exceptions (see for example Dewing 2007; Sabat 2005) little focus has been placed on understanding how issues of capacity and competence influence how one views oneself, interacts with one's world and is treated by others. Yet, as Sabat (2005) notes, the risks of 'excess disability' – disability that is rooted in the social world rather than the brain of the person with dementia – is high when someone is constructed as 'dysfunctional'. Thus, the need to examine decision-making within the context of a personhood lens has the potential to make unique contributions for understanding both the dementia experience and capacity issues in general.

When this lens is brought in to understand issues associated with decision-making in the area of dementia, a unique set of questions emerge that have yet to be addressed. At a broad level, how is the notion of capacity, or incapacity, incorporated into a more holistic understanding and treatment of the person with dementia? In particular, how can the relationship between personhood, dementia and decision-making ability be conceptualized and understood? Where do notions of capacity fit, particularly when premised upon cognitive functioning? Much of the literature has considered capacity only in relation to formal aspects of living; how relevant is this concept for understanding the more informal, everyday activities of the person with dementia? Arguably, it is at this level that most decision-making activity occurs, yet there is a paucity of research focused on fleshing out these day-to-day decision-making processes. What is the interplay between capacity and personhood in decision-making at the individual, familial, community and socio-political level?

More specifically, when capacity is compromised, how can the person with dementia be involved in his or her own care? There is a growing body of research that highlights the need to 'hear the voice' of the individual with dementia, but what this looks like and how it can be done when the person is considered 'incapable' is unclear. Taken a step further, what does the decision-making process look like when one person has a dementia that renders him or her cognitively unable to understand or appreciate significant aspects of a decision? Legislation such as England's Mental Capacity Act 2005 is designed to promote autonomy even for people lacking capacity. How will this be achieved? More specifically, how do family members and other relational partners respond? Little attention has been given to teasing out the complexities associated with the transference of power related to decision-making. A social constructionist account of personhood would suggest that this is a critical area for better understanding when someone has dementia.

Combined, these questions suggest the need for an approach to understanding decisional capacity in persons with dementia that is much more holistic, dynamic and interactive. Traditional ways of addressing these issues have typically precluded developing this more complex, textured understanding. Rather, understanding of these issues has often been discipline-specific with few attempts to overlap. In particular, much of the research is legally or biomedically based with almost no references to the social approaches to care that are beginning to dominate the dementia literature. Moye and colleagues (2007) recognize the ineffectiveness of this, noting the communication breakdown between different disciplines – particularly the legal and health professionals – and calling for a conceptual framework that will promote dialogue.

As one way of beginning this dialogue, an international, interdisciplinary workshop, led by researchers at the Centre for Research on Personhood in Dementia (CRPD), was held in Vancouver in May 2007.[1] The intent of the workshop was to begin a discussion that would lead to the development of a multi-layered approach for understanding decision-making in dementia that integrated ideas from a variety of perspectives, including legal, ethical, biomedical, psychosocial and environmental. Specific questions guiding the two days of discussion included: How do issues of decision-making influence the experience of living with dementia for the person with dementia and his or her significant others? How do formal and informal assessments of capacity/incapacity integrate notions of personhood? How can the personhood of the individual with dementia be respected, even in situations where decisional competence is challenged and/or removed? How does the organizational culture of dementia care impact understanding of decision-making? How is this different across cultures?

OVERVIEW OF THIS BOOK

This book comes out of these discussions. As a first step in preparing for the workshop, each participant was invited to prepare a position paper describing a particular issue related to the interface between personhood and decision-making in dementia – no further specifications were given. A website was established so that all participants could preview these position papers prior to the workshop. These then formed the foundation for two days of discussions. Following the workshop, participants were invited to contribute chapters based on their initial position papers. The result is a range of papers compiled in this volume that demonstrates the rich and varied way that this interface can be approached. The volume is unique in its efforts to draw in perspectives from the social sciences, health sciences and legal domains in order to promote a more integrated discussion.

The papers are organized into three sections: exploring ways of conceptualizing the issues, examining practice and policy issues, and uncovering the complexities associated with day-to-day decision-making across the dementia trajectory.

Part 1 lays the foundation for later chapters by examining the notion of personhood and beginning to conceptualize how theoretical and philosophical issues associated with personhood may inform our understanding of decision-making in the dementia experience. The intent was to extend conventional ideas about personhood, decision-making and dementia by introducing a variety of alternative ways for thinking about these issues. Drawing on a diverse range of interdisciplinary and international perspectives, this section explores philosophical, cultural and moral aspects of personhood and decision-making in dementia. It begins with Baldwin's discussion of personhood and decision-making in dementia within the theoretical framework of narrative, presenting a view of personhood not as a particular status, but rather as narrative process. He then draws on narrative theory to explore how concepts such as emplotment and narrative agency can be used in decision-making to optimize continuity of the trajectory of a person's narrative. In the next chapter, Smith introduces a sociological perspective on autonomy, contextualizing it within the social practices that define both its nature and the circumstances under which it can be compromised. Drawing on Bourdieu's concepts of habitus and symbolic capital, he explores decision-making in dementia in terms of both cultural notions of personhood and institutional imperatives in modern health care. Harrigan and Gillett in Chapter 4 develop these themes further, exploring how negative influences of modernity on the concept of person, which are particularly undermining for those with dementia, can be countered by notions of more narratively situated relational selves. In the fifth chapter, Tsai extends this discussion in a new direction, describing how Confucian conceptions of 'persons', which include both autonomous and relational dimensions of personhood, can influence decision-making for persons with dementia. In the final chapter of Part 1, Hulko and Stern pick up the theme of cultural interpretations of personhood and autonomy as they examine how these notions are problematic in decision-making for persons with dementia when viewed in the context of cultural difference and cultural safety. With its discussion of two case studies illustrating these tensions, as well as the authors' attention to implications for practice, this chapter begins to move the focus from conceptual formulations to discussions of social policy and practice.

The focus on social policy and practice is picked up in Part 2. Combined, the chapters in this section present an international overview of some of the current issues and developments related to understanding and evaluating capacity of individuals who have dementia. Bringing in an English perspective, Manthorpe examines the new Mental Capacity Act 2005, focusing in particular on how it interacts with a move toward greater personalization of social care in England and Wales for managing risk, protection and autonomy with vulnerable populations. Her discussion highlights the implications of this interaction, including its impact on person-centred practice, for all those involved in decision-making with persons with dementia in the provision of social care and other services. In Chapter 8, the discussion moves to a Canadian context as O'Connor and Donnelly shift the focus from a legislative approach to examine clinical practices in assessing and determining capacity for older adults with dementia in a context of abuse. They highlight limitations associated with the focus on cognitive functioning that characterizes current practices for assessing capacity. Hall then moves the discussion from clinical practice to law as she explores legal interpretations of capacity, vulnerability, risk and consent, focusing in particular on undue influence and unconscionability. She highlights the potential importance of these latter constructs as a means for shifting the focus from individual deficiency associated with capacity to situational judgements. In the final chapter of this section, Tilse, Wilson and Setterlund draw on Australian policy and practice to examine decision-making regarding finances as a key area where older people with dementia can be either included or excluded. Drawing on their research around asset management, they identify how a personhood approach can be promoted to include persons with dementia in financial decision-making.

Part 3 moves into the uncharted terrain of considering how decision-making and personhood issues are addressed in the day-to-day experience of living with dementia. The intent of this section is to begin to capture the unique issues that underpin informal decision-making across a variety of settings (home, community and institutions) and points in the illness trajectories. Where Part 1 is largely conceptual and Part 2 is more practice-based, Part 3 presents new research being undertaken in this area. Keady, Williams and Hughes-Roberts begin this investigation by exploring the inter-relationship of biography, coping/adaptive strategies and day-to-day decision-making for persons with dementia following their diagnosis of Alzheimer disease. This qualitative multiple-case study demonstrates how individual decisions about seeking a diagnosis can only be understood in the context of each person's ways of living day-to-day. In the next chapter, O'Connor and Kelson use an indepth case study of a woman with dementia and her husband to capture the dynamic, complex nature of the decision-making process around the decision to use support services. Their research draws attention to the pivotal role played by the person with dementia in this decision, irrespective of cognitive capacity. In Chapter 13, Purves and Perry draw on the analysis of one family's conversations to examine how family members support – or fail to support – involvement of the person with dementia in everyday decision-making. Finally, Kontos and Naglie move from the community setting into the institution, using the notion of embodied selfhood to extend the discussion of decision-making to considerations of persons with very advanced dementia. Drawing on findings from focus groups of practitioners in long-term care, they explore how bodily movements and gestures represent socio-cultural self-expressions, informing a process of clinical decision-making that can take into account the particularities and individuality of a person with dementia, even when that person's cognitive abilities are severely compromised. Combined, these chapters begin to tease out the nuances, contradictions and complexities inherent in a relational approach to understanding decision-making.

These chapters represent diverse disciplinary perspectives and approaches to understanding the interface between personhood, dementia and decision-making. Taken together, they offer a unique opportunity to explore how differences and congruencies across these perspectives can inform our understanding of this conceptual interface. Accordingly, the final chapter is an integrative commentary which highlights the dominant, cross-cutting themes and identifies next steps for research, social policy and clinical practice.

ENDNOTE

1.   Further details about this workshop can be found at http://crpd.swfs.ubc.ca/ decision-making-workshop.

REFERENCES

Bartlett, R. and O'Connor, D. (2007) 'From personhood to citizenship: Broadening the lens for dementia practice and research.' *Journal of Aging Studies 21*, 2, 107–118.

Bond, J., Corner, L., Lilley, A. and Ellwood, C. (2002) 'Medicalization of insight and caregivers' response to risk in dementia.' *Dementia 1*, 3, 313–328.

Boyle, G. (2008) 'The Mental Capacity Act 2005: Promoting the citizenship of people with dementia?' *Health and Social Care in the Community 16*, 5, 529–537.

Buchanan, A. and Brock, D. (1989) *Deciding for Others: The Ethics of Surrogate Decision-Making.* Cambridge and New York: Cambridge University Press.

Cheston, R. and Bender, M. (1999) *Understanding Dementia: The Man with the Worried Eyes.* London: Jessica Kingsley Publishers.

Clare, L., Rowlands, J., Bruce, E., Surr, C. and Downs, M. (2008) '"I don't do like I used to do": A grounded theory approach to conceptualizing awareness in people with moderate to severe dementia living in long-term care.' *Social Science and Medicine 66*, 11, 2366–2377.

Cohen, D. and Eisdorfer, C. (1986) *The Loss of Self.* New York and London: W.W. Norton.

Dewing, J. (2007) 'Participatory research: A method for process consent with persons who have dementia.' *Dementia 6*, 1, 11–25.

Harding, N. and Palfrey, C. (1997) *The Social Construction of Dementia.* London: Jessica Kingsley Publishers.

Harrison, C. (1993) 'Personhood, dementia and integrity of a life.' *Canadian Journal on Aging 12*, 4, 428–440.

Kitwood, T. (1997) *Dementia Reconsidered: The Person Comes First.* Buckingham: Open University Press.

Kluge, E.H.W. (2005) 'Competence, capacity, and informed consent: Beyond the cognitive-competence model.' *Canadian Journal on Aging 24*, 3, 295–304.

Marson, D.C. and Briggs, S.D. (2001) 'Assessing Competency in Alzheimer's Disease: Treatment Consent Capacity and Financial Capacity.' In S. Gauthier and J. Cummings (eds) *Alzheimer's Disease.* London: J. Martin Dunitz.

Moye, J. and Marson, D.C. (2007) 'Assessment of decision-making capacity in older adults: An emerging area of practice and research.' *Journal of Gerontology Series B: Psychological Sciences and Social Sciences 62B*, 1, P3–P11.

Moye, J., Butz, S.W., Marson, D.C., Wood, E. and the ABA-APA Capacity Assessment of Older Adults Working Group (2007) 'A conceptual model and assessment template for capacity evaluation in adult guardianship.' *The Gerontologist 47*, 5, 591–603.

Nolan, M.R., Lundh, U., Grant, G. and Keady, J. (eds) (2003) *Partnerships in Family Care: Understanding the Caregiving Career.* Maidenhead: Open University Press.

Post, S.G. (2000) 'The Concept of Alzheimer Disease in a Hypercognitive Society.' In P.J. Whitehouse, K. Maurer and J.F. Ballenger (eds) *Concepts of Alzheimer Disease: Biological, Clinical, and Cultural Perspectives.* Baltimore, MD: Johns Hopkins University Press.

Royall, D.R. (2002) 'Back to the future of mental capacity assessment.' *Journal of the American Geriatrics Society 50*, 11, 1884–1885.

Sabat, S. (2005) 'Capacity for decision-making in Alzheimer's disease: Selfhood, positioning and semiotic people.' *Australian and New Zealand Journal of Psychiatry 39*, 11–12, 1030–1035.

Shulman, K.I., Cohen, C.A. and Hull, I. (2005) 'Psychiatric issues in retrospective challenges of testamentary capacity.' *International Journal of Geriatric Psychiatry 20*, 1, 63–69.

Woods, B. and Pratt, R. (2005) 'Awareness in dementia: Ethical and legal issues in relation to people with dementia.' *Aging and Mental Health 9*, 5, 423–429.

PART 1

Conceptualizing
the Issues

CHAPTER 2

Narrative and Decision-Making

CLIVE BALDWIN

It is nowadays commonplace to state the importance of narrative in under-standing the lives of others. For some, narrative gives a peculiar insight into the reality of others' lives that enhances our understanding; for others, narrative constitutes that reality. This is a distinction I want to hold on to from the outset in my exploration of decision-making in dementia care. The first position views narrative as a source of data to inform decision-making: the more information we have, the more likely we are to make good decisions (see e.g. Arras 1997; Charon 1994; Tomlinson 1997). This I term *narratively informed decision-making*. The second position – which I shall term *narrative decision-making* – regards narrative as central to the decision-making process: employing narrative concepts such as emplotment, characterization, narrative agency, narrative con-sistency and coherency and readership to structure decision-making. Here I will explore narrative decision-making as it might be applied in dementia care.

A NARRATIVE APPROACH TO PERSONHOOD

The issue of personhood is an important one in dementia care – to what extent does personhood remain intact with the onset and progression of dementia? Opinion is divided with well-respected authors on both sides of the debate: those who would argue that personhood is diminished or lost in dementia (e.g. Brock 1993) and those that it remains (e.g. Kitwood 1997). The issue turns, I believe, on how we view personhood: authors such as Brock viewing it as residing in cognitive agency, those such as Kitwood as being attributable to each and every human being regardless of ability. Here I want to suggest that personhood is more a process – and a narrative process at that – to which we all contribute.

The view that we are narrative beings is well argued by authors such as Alisdair MacIntyre (1984), Jerome Bruner (1987) and Charles Taylor (1989). For these authors, among others, not only do we exist in a story-telling world but our very Selves are constituted by the stories we and others tell about ourselves. Our experience (of both the world and ourselves) is not reality given narrative form but rather our narrative form made real. In other words, we are our stories – to be unheard, unrecognized, unremembered is, according to Bakhtin (1984), absolute death. In these stories we constitute ourselves as persons in accordance with concepts of ourselves. These self-concepts are not static, and our identity is a combination of historical narrative and literary fiction. What flows from this is that narrativity – and thus personhood – is a performative activity. Such activity requires agency and opportunity. In what follows, I will discuss five aspects of narrative theory that are pertinent to the narrative Self and narrative agency and conclude with some comment about the implications of these for decision-making in dementia care.

FIVE ASPECTS OF NARRATIVE THEORY

In my pursuit of narrative decision-making, I want to put forward five inter-related aspects of narrative theory for consideration:

- genre
- character and role
- narrative agency
- narrative consistency and coherency
- readership.

These essential features of narrative are what distinguish narrative decision-making from decision-making that is simply informed by narratives.

Genre

Life is made up of a series of stories, somehow linked together. The bringing together of a series of stories into a larger story is the location of those stories within a specific genre that helps make sense of those stories. Traditionally there are fundamentally four story-types (adapted from Boje 2001):

- *Romance* – a drama of self-identification symbolized by a hero's (or heroine's) victory over the world of experience. A good example of romantic is the quest narrative, a heroic journey. The hero is redeemed and/or liberated.

- *Satire (irony)* – the opposite of Romance, a drama of apprehension symbolized by the hero's captivity in the world. The hero is never able to overcome the darkness, get out of the abyss. Irony of situation – discrepancy between appearance and reality, or between expectation and fulfilment, or between what is and what would seem appropriate.

- *Tragedy* – the hero is defeated by the experiences of the world, yet hope exists for those left behind by their understanding of the limits of overcoming the abyss. Liberation is possible, but the hero falls into the abyss.

- *Comedy* – there is hope for the hero in a temporary triumph over darkness. Comedy offers temporary reconciliation or harmony. Reconciliations are symbolized by a festive occasion, and harmony can be achieved between conflicting parties. The essential difference between tragedy and comedy is in the depiction of human nature: tragedy shows greatness in human nature and human freedom, whereas comedy shows human weakness and human limitation. The purpose of comedy is to make us laugh and, at the same time, to help to illuminate human nature and human weaknesses. Conventionally comedies have a happy ending.

These four are not the only possible genres (and indeed are peculiar to the Western tradition) but are presented here as illustrative of how the frame of a narrative or series of narratives can bring meaning to those narratives. For example, *Love Story* (1970, Arthur Hiller) is the story of star-crossed lovers who face adversity, firstly in the form of parental disapproval and finally in Jenny's terminal illness. The story makes sense because it is, essentially, a tragedy. Trying to understand *Love Story* as satire would simply confuse. Similarly, in *Stranger than Fiction* (2006, Marc Forster), the protagonist, Harold Crick, starts to hear an external narration of his life as he lives it (for example, while brushing his teeth he hears a narrator saying that Harold Crick brushed his teeth the same way every day). The ongoing external narration prompts Harold to seek advice, initially from a psychiatrist who diagnoses schizophrenia, but latterly from a professor of literature who informs Harold that if this experience is to make sense Harold needs to work out what sort of story it is – a comedy or tragedy. Only by doing so will Harold understand his own life.

Character and role

Narratives are populated by characters – some major players, some bit players, some walk-on parts. Some contribute greatly to the impetus of the story, others very little, if at all. Sometimes characters will be foregrounded as others recede into the background. In thinking about characters and roles, we need to be aware of the various ways they can affect narratives.

- The decisions characters make help set the trajectory of who they become – for example, in *Unforgiven* (1992, Clint Eastwood), Bill Munny inexorably returns to his past as a vicious, violent gunslinger through a series of decisions that set that trajectory. And again, Phil Connors, played by Bill Murray, in *Groundhog Day* (1993, Harold Ramis) is forced to live out the same day again and again until, through changing his decisions and actions in that one day, he becomes a model citizen; or Mona Bergeron in *Vagabonde* (1985, Agnes Varda) in which, having started with Mona being found frozen to death, a series of interviews with secondary characters charts her last few months with each event and decision being, in hindsight, a clear marker of the trajectory towards a lonely and unwitnessed death.

- Minor characters can substantially affect the outcome of the narrative; for example, the angel warning the magi not to report the whereabouts of Jesus' birth to Herod.

- Different characters have different interests and different preferred narrative trajectories. For example, consider the case of Dax Cowart (Kliever 1989): Dax himself, having suffered extreme burns in a propane accident, wished to terminate his narrative through being allowed to die; his mother, a committed Christian, did not see this trajectory as acceptable as her son had not made peace with God; a number of his doctors wanted to 'save' Dax and thus prove the efficacy of their profession.

It is my contention that a fundamental aspect of narrative decision-making is the import ascribed to any character or role. In healthcare interactions, for example, often much weight is given to the advice or opinion of health professionals. While this is, on one level, not surprising (after all they are more knowledgeable), they are, in the narrative scheme of things, relatively minor players and, unlike the angel in the nativity story, not messengers from God. Most healthcare interactions, even ones that concern ongoing conditions such as dementia, are, I believe, minor points in a much broader and longer narrative. The questions for decision-making are what import should be given to what are essentially bit players and whether or not the broader and longer narrative should be subsumed by decisions made in such episodic encounters.

Narrative agency

Narrative agency is an essential part of being a narrative Self. It is both the ability and opportunity to construct one's own narrative, and also the opportunity to contribute to the narratives of others. The narrative agency of people with dementia is constrained in two main ways: the exclusionary nature of linguistic/narrative convention and the limited opportunities for narrativity. These constraints are not necessarily the result of the dementia but rather the limits of narrativity imposed upon those living with dementia. Each constraint can be overcome by reconceptualizing the issue, thus opening a space for people with dementia to participate in the narrative enterprise.

The first of these linguistic conventions that set the boundaries of what is recognized as narrative exclude those who cannot conform to those conventions, such as those living with dementia when use of language is compromised. To express oneself narratively requires a degree of conformity to narrative rules or habits or customs. Adherence to such rules might vary in degree but it becomes apparent that beyond a certain threshold 'differences of degree effectively become differences of kind; beyond that point a sequence may begin to display so little narrativity that it can no longer be processed as a story at all' (Herman 2002, p.100). Consider the following from Herman (2002):

1. A bad man walked in. Then a beneficent sorcerer pulled the lever, and the bad man was instantaneously inebriated.

2. A splubba walked in. A gingy beebed the yuck, and the splubba was orped.

3. Oe splubba fibblo. Sim oe gingy beebie ca yuck, i ca splubba orpa.

The first of these is easily and straightforwardly recognizable as a narrative. The second, while unintelligible in terms of what actually happened and to whom or what, is recognizable as a narrative: first this happened, then that. The third displays little if any narrativity because it 'lacks sufficient grammatical structure for recipients to infer actants and entities populating a story world' (Herman 2002, p.102).

For those living with dementia the difficulties encountered with expressive language and loss of memory for recent events and disorientation to place and time may limit the possibility of engaging narratively with the world and with others. Utterances may appear to others as lacking in meaning due to the person's difficulty in retrieving the correct word from memory or difficulty with putting words in the correct sequence along with the mis-identification and difficulty in retrieving the characters, events or context. If one expects a higher degree of conformity to narrative rules, habits or customs, then it is possible that one would see people living with dementia as losing narrative agency sooner rather than later.

Stories can also be articulated as much through dance, movement and artistic expression as through language – if we, as readers, are sensitive enough to the narrative features of such media – and this is, of course, a familiar and common approach in the arts. Similarly, Downs, Small and Froggatt (2006) cite literature from Norberg and colleagues demonstrating the effectiveness of communication styles including affirmation, confirmation and communion. They also cite the growing use of sound, music, dance and movement in making contact. People living with dementia may find (and/or need to be encouraged to find) non-verbal means of expressing their narrative agency. This in turn requires a level of narrative literacy (i.e. the ability to recognize the narrative aspects of non-verbal expression) on the part of those who care.

The other element of narrative agency, as I have defined it here, is having the opportunity to express oneself narratively. People living with dementia, however, find themselves narratively constrained in two ways. First, opportunities for narrative expression are limited: people living with dementia may experience a loss of control, in that decisions are made for them (and stories made about them) as they are increasingly defined as lacking capacity, and a loss of narrative opportunity because of lessened opportunity for social interaction. Second, the mental space within which narratives can be told is constrained through the mobilization of the meta-narrative of dementia, which defines the person in terms of decline, loss and fragmented cognitive functioning (and thus less able to tell a recognizable narrative) and the recuperation of expressions of agency (such as 'wandering', 'challenging behaviour', 'fidgeting') as symptomatic of the dementia itself (see Kitwood 1997).

The second constraint on the narrative agency of people living with dementia is the limited opportunities provided to contribute to the narrative of others. Involved as we are in a web of stories (webs of interlocution as Taylor 1989 puts it) – that we tell and that are told about us – our narrative agency spills over from the stories we tell into the contribution we make to the stories of others.

In *In the Vineyard of the Text*, Illich (1996) makes a distinction between monastic and scholastic reading. Monastic reading, Illich says, was an embodied activity that required the reader to incorporate the reading into one's own life. The text was something that was approached as having something to say directly to one's own experience and existence ('What does this text say to my life?'). Over the course of history, around the 12th century, monastic reading was replaced by what Illich calls scholastic reading. This form of reading, brought about by physical changes in the text such as spaces, paragraphs, punctuation and so on, came to focus on what the text itself was saying and thus the text became an object in its own right and a subject of debate ('What is this text saying?' Or 'What is the correct reading of this text?').

I want to suggest that a monastic approach to reading the text of another's life restores some degree of narrative agency to that person and thus displays more narrative probity than a scholastic reading that distances the other's narrative. In answering the question 'What does this narrative say to and about my own life?' we are opening the door for others to contribute meaningfully and deeply to the construction of our life narratives. With regard to people living with dementia, all too often the narrative flow is one way – from the professional to the person with dementia. We focus on what 'we' can do in 'their' lives and fail to appreciate what 'they' do in ours. For example, many carers I have interviewed have reported that through the caring experience they have developed patience, tolerance and a sense of immediacy, all due to the presence in their lives of a relative with dementia – or have had to think carefully and considerately about their relationships, their approach to truth-telling and their ability to inhabit a moral world when previously taken-for-granted values and frameworks are challenged or undermined by the onset and progression of dementia. In these ways, the narrative agency of those living with dementia is maintained through the contribution they make to the lives of others.

Narrative consistency and coherency

Another aspect of narrativity that is relevant to decision-making in dementia care is a focus on narrative consistency and coherency; that is, the maintenance of the historical continuity of backdrop, story and protagonist. In dementia it is often argued that there is a split between the historical self and the demented self, that the demented self is different from the previous self. We do not need to think of the Self in dementia, however, in these 'then' and 'now' terms, for this is biographically disruptive. It is not unlike Gregor Samsa in Kafka's *Metamorphosis* (1916) who wakes up one morning to find himself transformed into an insect. Dementia is a lived process in which the Self may change.

Two things are required to maintain consistency and coherency in this process of change: first, an understanding of the present in the context of the past (as illustrated by the following story); second, the formulation and maintenance of a trajectory that emerges from the backdrop.

A gentleman in a nursing home would take all his clothes off in the sitting room every afternoon and the staff would scurry around collecting his socks and his trousers and things. This behaviour, while appearing odd, makes perfect sense against the narrative backdrop of the gentleman having been a rower at university in his youth. Every day in the afternoon – because there would be no lectures in the afternoons – he would be stripping off and going off to practise on the river.

Hogeway, a residential community in the Netherlands for people with dementia, embodies this second requirement, providing care on the basis of seven different lifestyles that are, in turn, based on a detailed study of cultural patterns and practices across the Netherlands. Each group within Hogeway has its own pattern of daily life and activities that reflects what, for them, are the ordinary, everyday lives that individuals would have lived when in the community. Individuals are assessed and placed in the lifestyle group that most closely matches their pre-admission life: emphasis is placed on establishing the type of work they did, their religious beliefs, their social class, their cultural patterns and practices, their hobbies and interests, and on finding ways to facilitate activities which help to keep them anchored in reality. This is more than simply understanding individual lives; it is maintaining those lives into the future, as far as is possible (see Notter, Spijker and Stomp 2004).

In maintaining narrative consistency and coherency, we are locating people within the wider narratives of their lives (and the lives of others). Such narratives allow for both continuity and change; continuity contributing towards security, attachment, a sense of home and so on, change contributing to the ongoing becoming and creativity of being human. This narrative consistency and continuity helps ground decision-making within the wider lives of people living with dementia, avoiding some of the difficulties posed by the debate about the 'then' and 'now' self, and helps to maintain the integrity of the persons by limiting the disruption caused by changing circumstances.

Readership

Finally in our consideration of narrativity and decision-making comes the issue of readership. Just as we author our stories, we also read or listen to the stories of Others. Reading and listening are not neutral or distanced activities, but positioned and involved. Let me tell you a story (adapted from Booth 2001):

One time there were two farmers that lived out on the road to Carico. They were always good friends, and Bill's eldest boy had been seeing one of Sam's daughters. Everything was going fine till the morning they met down by the creek, and Sam was pretty goddam mad. 'Bill,' says he, 'from now on I don't want that boy of yours to set foot on my place.' 'Why, what's he done?' asked the boy's daddy.

'He pissed in the snow, that's what he done, right in front of my house!'

'But surely, there ain't no great harm in that,' Bill says.

'No harm!' hollered Sam. 'Hell's fire, he pissed so it spelled Lucy's name, right there in the snow!'

'The boy shouldn't have done that,' says Bill. 'But I don't see nothing so terrible bad about it.'

'Well, by God, I do!' yelled Sam. 'There was two sets of tracks! And besides, don't you think I know my own daughter's hand-writing?'

Our responses to the story – whether we laughed, were puzzled or offended (or any other response) – indicate two things: first, that we brought something of ourselves to the reading or hearing of that story; and, second, the extent to which we aligned ourselves with the implied audience of the story (i.e. those who understand the innuendo and find the story funny). The first reflects our position (whether real or idealized); the second, our involvement.

It is not a matter of choosing whether or not to be involved in the story – simply by the fact of our readership we are involved – but of choosing *how* to be involved. In writing about Native American stories, Thomas King (2005) suggests at the end of each chapter that what readers do with the story is up to them; they can re-tell it, they can work with it, they can adapt it, they can ignore it – what they cannot do is say that they never heard it.

Our choice of response is thus a function of our character: '...the kinds of decisions we confront, indeed the very way we describe a situation, is a function of the kind of character we have' (Hauerwas 1977, p.20). Character, according to Hauerwas, is forged not through adherence to abstract principles or theories but by the stories of which we are a part and which form the milieu in which we live our lives. These stories tie together the contingencies that make up our lives and set the context for our moral judgement. Narrative, readership and character are all intertwined in our decision-making. Thus, when we make decisions with or for people living with dementia, how we do this reflects and constitutes the sort of people we are, and are becoming. Decision-making is thus not a neutral act but one integrally entwined with ethics and thus with character.

NARRATIVE DECISION-MAKING

At this point, even if you have some sympathy with my approach, you may be thinking what any of this has to do with decision-making. In brief, if we are to take a narrative approach to decision-making, we need to formulate decisions that:

- are in keeping with the type of story it is (genre)
- are in keeping with the characters and their respective roles (character and characterization), perhaps acknowledging the often relative unimportance of professionals in the narratives of people living with dementia (after all, professionals are oft-times episodic minor characters in life)
- facilitate narrative agency (authorship) – through extending our understandings of narrative, narrativizing other symbolic forms of expression or co-construction of narratives (see Keady and Williams 2005)
- move forward the story (plot trajectory, consistency and coherency), linguistically in the stories we tell, socially in the relationships we create and maintain, and culturally in the environments we create
- are in accordance with who we want to become (readership) – our decisions and character being intertwined (see Hauerwas 1977).

If we are to succeed in doing the above, we need to develop our narrative literacy – for example, in determining what sort of story we are telling or is being told (see Harold Crick above). In addition to developing an understanding of the five aspects of narrativity outlined above, it will also be necessary to develop a stock of stories on which to draw (both in and across genres). Stories are understood in relation to other stories (relating both to the individual and the wide world) and the wider the range we have to draw upon, the more likely we are to be able to respond flexibly and appropriately:

> The person with moderate or moderately severe dementia may be able to present only fragments of a performance story. The more a nurse knows

about narrative components or the different sections of a story, the more easily he or she can identify and follow up on a story fragment offered by a person with dementia. (Moore and Davis 2002, p.263)

This narrative literacy would involve the development of skills in examining the types and roles of narratives in the life of the person with dementia and looking to the construction of meaningful narratives for and with that person. For example, a narrative approach to the palliative care of persons with dementia might ask what narratives are in play in the situation (personal, institutional, discoursal), what the desired narrative trajectory is and how the chosen narrative maintains and develops the Self (see Baldwin 2006 for a description of what a narrative approach to palliative care might look like).

CONCLUDING REMARKS

Narrative decision-making stands in contrast to narratively informed decision-making. The former reaches deeper into the lives of those concerned and produces, maintains and manifests a continuity of trajectory that the latter can only mimic. To be sure, narratives are elicited in both approaches and both require sensitivity to the flux of narrativity. The difference lies in what is then done with those narratives. The former folds them back into the narrative enterprise, returning them to the context and dynamics from which they arose. The latter uses the elicited narratives to inform a different decision-making framework in order to make decisions about the context from which the narratives emerged. I am aware that much work needs to be done on developing a framework for narrative decision-making – I hope that this chapter is a useful and stimulating start.

REFERENCES

Arras, J.D. (1997) 'Nice Story, But So What? Narrative and Justification in Ethics.' In H.L. Nelson (ed.) *Stories and Their Limits: Narrative Approaches to Bioethics.* London: Routledge.

Bakhtin, M. (1984) *Problems of Dostoevsky's Poetics.* Translated by C. Emerson. Minneapolis, MN: University of Minnesota Press.

Baldwin, C. (2006) 'Narrative Ethics and Ethical Narratives in Dementia.' In A. Burns and B. Winblad (eds) *Severe Dementia.* London: Wiley.

Boje, D.M. (2001) *Narrative Methods for Organizational and Communication Research.* London: Sage.

Booth, W.C. (2001) 'Literary criticism and the pursuit of character.' *Literature and Medicine* 20, 2, 97–108.

Brock, D.W. (1993) *Life and Death: Philosophical Essays in Biomedical Ethics.* Cambridge: Cambridge University Press.

Bruner, J.S. (1987) 'Life as narrative.' *Social Research 54,* 11–32.

Charon, R. (1994) 'Narrative Contributions to Medical Ethics: Recognition, Formulation, Interpretation, and Validation in the Practice of the Ethicist.' In E.R. DuBose, R. Hamel and L.J. O'Connell (eds) *A Matter of Principles? Ferment in U.S. Bioethics.* Valley Forge, PA: Trinity Press International.

Downs, M., Small, N. and Froggatt, K. (2006) 'Person-Centred Care for People with Severe Dementia.' In A. Burns and B. Winblad (eds) *Severe Dementia.* London: Wiley.

Hauerwas, S. with Bondi, R. and Burrell, D.B. (1977) *Truthfulness and Tragedy: Further Investigations into Christian Ethics.* London: University of Notre Dame Press.

Herman, D. (2002) *Story Logic: Problems and Possibilities of Narrative.* Lincoln, NE: University of Nebraska Press.

Illich, I. (1996) *In the Vineyard of the Text: A Commentary to Hugh's Didascalicon.* Chicago, IL: University of Chicago Press.

Karka, F. (1916) *The Metamorphosis.* Translated by Ian Johnstone (2009). Available at http://records.viu.ca/~johnstoi/stories/kafka-E.htm, accessed on 26 March 2009.

Keady, J. and Williams, S. (2005) 'Co-constructed inquiry: A new approach to the generation of shared knowledge in chronic illness.' RCN International Research Conference, Belfast, 8–11 March 2005.

King, T. (2005) *The Truth about Stories: A Native Narrative.* Minneapolis, MN: University of Minnesota Press.

Kitwood, T. (1997) *Dementia Reconsidered: The Person Comes First.* Buckingham: Open University Press.

Kliever, L.D. (1989) *Dax's Case: Essays in Medical Ethics and Human Meaning.* Dallas, TX: Southern Methodist University Press.

MacIntyre, A. (1984) *After Virtue: A Study in Moral Theory.* Notre Dame, IN: University of Notre Dame Press.

Moore, L.A. and Davis, B. (2002) 'Quilting narrative: Using repetition techniques to help elderly communicators.' *Geriatric Nursing 23,* 5, 262–266.

Notter, J., Spijker, T. and Stomp, K. (2004) 'Taking the community into the home.' *Health and Social Care in the Community 12,* 5, 448–453.

Taylor, C. (1989) *Sources of the Self.* Cambridge: Cambridge University Press.

Tomlinson, T. (1997) 'Perplexed about Narrative Ethics.' In H.L. Nelson (ed.) *Stories and Their Limits: Narrative Approaches to Bioethics.* London: Routledge.

CHAPTER 3

Decision-Making as Social Practice

Exploring the Relevance of Bourdieu's Concepts of Habitus and Symbolic Capital

ANDRÉ SMITH

INTRODUCTION

The issue of decision-making in dementia care has been predominantly investigated in terms of cognitive capacity and as a technical challenge of psychometric measurement (e.g. Fillenbaum, Landerman and Simonsick 1998; Lai and Karlawish 2007; Marson *et al.* 1994; Moye and Marson 2007). Capacity is presumed to decline more or less linearly with the loss of memory and decline in executive functions (Gurrera *et al.* 2007). In the end, individuals with dementia gradually lose the ability to make informed choices about matters of concern, including personal finances, self-care and decisions pertaining to medical treatment (Kim, Karlawish and Gurrera 2002). The social and ethical consequences of determining capacity have been well explored in the literature, particularly in terms of the potentially devastating consequences of underestimating decision-making capacity or failing to capture its more subtle and diverse expressions (Sabat 2005; Sadler, Bernstein and Marson 2003; Stewart 2006). However, what seems to be missing is a more contextualized reflection in relation to the social practices that define the nature of autonomy and the circumstances under which individuals with dementia lose the capacity to be the authors of their own destiny.

Decision-making relates to a fundamental debate in sociology – the relationship between agency and structure. Sociology has contributed a great deal of insight into the nature of this relationship, although theoretical traditions have historically focused on one or the other construct at the expense of understanding their interrelationship. Interpretive traditions like phenomenology and symbolic interactionism have generally reaffirmed the primacy of agency, proposing a view of structure as emerging from the meaning-making activities of social actors. By contrast, structuralist perspectives like functionalism and Marxism have privileged social structures in accounting for the ways actors fulfil their social roles or profit from one another. Criticisms of naivety and reductionism have been levelled at interpretive sociologists, while accusations of determinism have plagued structural sociologists. However, out of these debates have emerged useful compromises that offer a more synthetic view of agency and its relation to structure. One example is the sociology of Pierre Bourdieu. This chapter explores the applicability of Bourdieu's concepts of habitus and symbolic capital in understanding decision-making as a phenomenon rooted in cultural notions of personhood and mediated by the imperative of modern healthcare institutions to efficiently process individuals with diminished cognitive abilities.

HABITUS, FIELD AND CAPITAL

Bourdieu (1988) conceptualized habitus, field and capital as mechanisms involved in the reproduction of social class. These concepts are at the core of a sociology that unites social phenomenology and structuralism to explain the relationship between everyday practices and the context in which those practices take place. As Turner (1991) remarks, Bourdieu's sociology gives us 'a vision of social classes and the cultural forms associated with these classes' (p.512). From this perspective, social classes are understood in dynamic terms as fields of hierarchical positions structured by power relations, rules, rituals and conventions.

For Bourdieu, struggles over economic, social, cultural and symbolic forms of capital determine class structure. Those in the dominant class tend to possess the most (or most legitimized) forms of capital, whereas the lowest classes possess the least amount of capital, although there are corresponding similarities between, and within, different classes (Turner 1991). With the concept of habitus, Bourdieu explains how people learn to behave and represent the world in a manner consistent with their social class. He defines habitus as a system of personal dispositions that are constituted by lasting, acquired schemes of perception, thought and action (Turner 1991). Thus, habitus serves an instrumental function by transforming objective social structures into the subjective, mental experiences that social actors need to competently operate within the cultural fields to which they belong. By cultural field, Bourdieu means the 'institutions, rules, rituals, conventions, categories, designations and appointments which constitute an objective hierarchy, and which produce and authorize certain discourses and activities' (Webb, Schirato and Danaher 2002, pp.x–xi). The habitus explains how human action perpetuates these cultural fields through the 'unconscious internalization – particularly during early childhood – of objective chances that are common to members of a social class or status group' (Swartz 1997, p.104). Habitus thus 'represents a sort of deep-structuring cultural matrix that generates self-fulfilling prophecies according to different class opportunities' (*ibid.*). It is the internalization of success and failure that drives expectations and aspirations and reproduces class position through the behaviours of social actors. This process occurs below introspection and language as a form of knowledge learnt by the body and mind but not entirely articulated by social actors unless they confront situations that are highly regulated or that have explicit normative rules that supersede the influence of habitus. Bourdieu also conceptualizes habitus as a mechanism of social control that secures the complicity of social actors in their subordination. As Swartz (*ibid.*) puts it, habitus explains how social agents internalize structural disadvantages that then result in dispositions that continually produce self-defeating behaviours.

DEMENTIA AND THE FAILURE OF HABITUS

From a Bourdieuan perspective, dementia can be conceptualized as the failure of habitus. The disease is experienced as a gradual loss in the ability to assume the skills, habits, tastes and manners that signify one's position in a cultural field. Cognitive decline thus renders the habitus unintelligible to others. The consequences of this failure have been documented to some extent in the symbolic interactionist literature. For example, Sweeting and Gilhooly (1997) coin the term 'social death' in reference to how people with dementia are no longer responded to as human beings with moral status. Orona (1990) reports that family caregivers cope with the devastating impact of dementia by re-enacting life-long reciprocal patterns of interactions and behaviours with the demented relative, in a sense attempting to recreate the old habitus lost to the disease. In the same vein, Fontana and Smith (1989) discuss how family caregivers engage in remedial work to preserve the habitus, taking over the performance of familiar routines and activities to avoid being embarrassed by an affected relative in public situations. The authors query the usefulness of this remedial work when only 'remnants of the self' are present in the later stages of dementia (Fontana and Smith 1989, p.43). Finally, Blum (1991) focuses on the stigma associated with dementia behaviour, noting that family caregivers sometimes collude with others in the management impaired behaviour by identifying the presence of mental illness with the ubiquitous gesture of rotating the index finger by the side of the head.

These studies underline how the lack of intelligible habitus puts those with dementia at risk of being displaced from the cultural fields to which they belong by formal and family caregivers alike. For example, Bamford and Bruce (2000) report that what is said by persons with dementia tends to have little in common with what is reported by caregivers on measures used to evaluate the community services required by dementia sufferers. Similarly, Sands and collegues (2004) note the presence of considerable disagreement between how patients with Alzheimer's disease and their proxies rate quality of life. The unintelligibility of habitus is, in a sense, what is at the heart of what Kitwood (1988) calls a dialectical interplay between neuropathology and a social environment that can no longer make sense of the altered expression of the self. Like Bourdieu, Kitwood relies on social phenomenology when he describes the problem of dementia as one involving a 'disjunction between subjectivity and the social milieu in which subjectivity is maintained' (p.176). The theme of unintelligibility is also echoed by Sabat and Harré (1992) when they propose that the presumed loss of self in dementia should be seen as a consequence of distorted discursive practices and the unwillingness of others to relate to the self as expressed in the disease. They argue that the diminution in memory, information processing and word-finding abilities that characterize dementia result in the loss of a public form of the self. They describe this public self as a repertoire of personae selected so as to be recognized by others – a construct reminiscent of Bourdieu's habitus. This perspective is congruent with the notion of habitus as being situated within the individual but also ascribed by the collectivity of a cultural field.

In a heavily regulated society, the failure of habitus becomes a significant liability for individuals with dementia. It is not unusual for family members to describe the affected relative in terms of valued roles that can no longer be assumed: he was a great school teacher with a prodigious memory; she was a brilliant scientist; he was an attentive father; she was a caring mother; etc. Erasure of the habitus is further compounded by nihilistic portrayals of dementia in the media, for example 'the assassin of the mind', 'the long goodbye', 'the funeral that never ends', 'the death before death' and the 'silent epidemic' we are told that the disease 'steals the mind', 'makes shells of former selves' and results in 'the loss of self' (Gubrium 1986, p.119; Stafford 1992, p.167). Stafford (1992) p.167 refers to this process as a form of 'cultural coding', which he sees as mediating how affected individuals and their care-givers interpret the significance of memory loss, make decisions about seeking medical help and take actions about how to manage declining capacity.

This cultural coding of dementia needs to be understood in relation to notions of individualism and autonomy – which are viewed as foundational features of the self in Western culture. As Geertz (1973) states, the Western self is

> a bounded, unique, more or less integrated motivational and cognitive universe, a dynamic center of awareness, emotion, judgement, and action organized into a distinctive whole and set contrastively both against other such wholes and set against a social and natural background. (Cited in Csordas 1994, p.59)

This self belongs to a 'unified, coherent, and rational agent who is the author of his or her own experience and meaning' (Burr 1995, p.40). It expresses the presence of 'an autonomous entity defined by its distinctiveness and separate-ness from the natural and social world' (Chang 1988, p.186). Historically, the emergence of the individualistic self traces its roots back to the transformation of European society into an increasingly secular universe following the spread of Protestantism and Descartes' influential epistemological dictum (*cogito ergo sum*) placing the capacity for knowledge in the mind rather than as a function of God's will and the Church (Lukes 1973). The individualistic self was further articulated in the philosophy of humanism, which held as essential the notion that human beings internally generate ideas about the world and that each person has a unique identity that stabilizes in adult years. Dumont (1985) also remarks that this conception of the self follows the rise of societies that have reaffirmed the supremacy of free enterprise, liberty and equality. The individu-alistic self achieves perhaps its fullest recognition in capitalist economies, where it is viewed as 'the actual or imminent realization of the final stage of human progress' (Lukes 1973, p.26).

The individualistic self is reaffirmed in everyday life through practices that signify one's separateness from others and society. As Chang (1988) remarks, these practices have become so embedded in the fabric of Western culture that they result in the perception of this self as being factual and universal. Only when contrasting the individualistic self to alternate conceptualizations does its cultural specificity become apparent. For example, as Landrine (1992) notes,

Eastern cultures generally have a more collective understanding of the self, which is seen as embedded in social interactions and relationships rather than as a separate entity existing independently from context. The self is also perceived more as a receptacle for the spirits of ancestors and other immaterial entities (Landrine 1992). In everyday life, this more collective self exists as the intersection of multiple relations with family, ancestors, community and religious traditions (Chang 1988).

Reflecting on the cultural relativity of the self allows us to examine more critically the approaches that are used to evaluate capacity in dementia. One can argue that such approaches rest on the notion that human beings exist as social agents only when they possess the capacity to engage in behaviour independently from the wishes of others and in independence from the institutions to which they belong. Psychometric assessments are thus designed to capture this individualistic performance of capacity, forgoing the possibility that individuals with dementia can operate as agents collectively defined at the nexus of supportive social relations. Sabat (2005) goes further by expressing concerns about the potential for current neuropsychological assessment practices to disadvantageously position people with dementia, thus undermining their rights to make their own decisions. He calls for revised practises that can take into account for the more subtle and complex manifestations of meaning-making ability and selfhood. Several other researchers have also called for the development of measures that give greater priority to personhood and subjective experience (Bamford and Bruce 2000; Merchant and Hope 2004; Whitlatch, Feinberg and Tucke 2005). However, these efforts can only be fully actualized once we interrogate the discourses of dementia that privilege individualizing notions of capacity, autonomy and independence.

THE SYMBOLIC VIOLENCE OF CLINICAL ASSESSMENT PRACTICES

Bourdieu challenges us to think about the relations of domination between individuals and their social institutions. While originally formulated as a critique of French class structure, Bourdieu's sociology has also important implications for analysing the power relations between individuals diagnosed with dementia and the institutions mandated to evaluate their cognitive capacity. This section examines the practices that govern the identification of the failing habitus, the manner in which those practices represent a struggle over desirable forms of symbolic capital, and the symbolic violence potentially engendered by such pursuits.

While economic capital is a common source of struggle, Bourdieu (1988) saw symbolic and cultural forms of capital as equally contested. Symbolic capital derives value from the prestige, honour and the right to be listened to in a given cultural field. Symbolic capital is closely associated with cultural capital, which refers to the competencies, skills and qualifications conferred to actors by their social institutions. Thus, actors who accumulate a great deal of cultural capital are more likely to occupy symbolically powerful positions in a field. The concept of symbolic capital is particularly useful in explaining the dynamics of power relations in organizations (Everett 2002). From a Bourdieuan perspective, the professional practices surrounding the assessment of capacity in dementia can be considered as 'struggles [that] take place over resources, stakes and access' (*ibid.*, p.62). More specifically, the social and economic capital invested in developing assessment tools gives researchers potential access to significant symbolic capital once a method or an instrument is scientifically validated. What is at stake here is prestige and the legitimacy to claim best practice.

However, the pursuit of symbolic capital increases the potential for what Bourdieu calls symbolic violence – a form of misrecognition (or misrepresentation) of oppressive power relations as natural features of the world. For Bourdieu, symbolic violence is perpetrated against vulnerable social groups by attributing to them inferior traits using social classifications that are misrepresented as naturalistic categories (e.g. gender, race, social class). Such misrecognition serves to justify oppressive practices – denying those groups access to resources and limiting their social mobility. In the case of dementia, an argument can be made that psychometric assessment technologies legitimize the traumatic processing of individuals with dementia in bureaucratized systems of care on the pretext of helping people who have lost the capacity to make their own decisions. These technologies expedite a passage into social irrelevance by permitting the removal of citizenship, justifying forced admission into exploitive and substandard care facilities, and facilitating the pharmacological control of legitimate expression of grief and protest. Kitwood (1990) also speaks of this symbolic violence when he describes as 'malignant social psychology' the manner in which formal caregivers exclude persons with dementia from meaningful social contact, causing hopelessness and depression that exacerbate the existing cognitive decline. He characterizes this malignant social psychology in terms of negative attitudes like disempowerment, infantilization, stigmatization, invalidation and banishment. These attitudes are fed by accepted notions that a socially meaningful self can only exist when high-level abilities such as rationality and intentionality are present (e.g. Beard 2004; Gubrium 1986).

The concept of symbolic violence draws attention to the importance of adopting more respectful conceptualizations of the self that offer the possibility of developing care interventions that positively influence the dementia experience. While the neuropathology of dementia cannot be reversed, positive social interventions can mitigate the extent of the disability (Harrison 1993; Kitwood and Bredin 1992; Miller *et al.* 2001), improve quality of life (Bamford and Bruce 2000; Golander and Raz 1996; Sabat and Harré 1992) and reduce the agitation and disruptive behaviours that make providing care so difficult (Matthews, Farrell and Blackmore 1996; Woods and Ashley 1995; Woods 2001).

CONCLUSION

Sabat and Harré (1992) argue that dementia should be understood as a problem of intelligibility rather than as one of inevitable erasure of the self. Bourdieu's sociology draws attention to how current clinical approaches for assessing decision-making capacity do little to improve intelligibility but rather tend to legitimize oppressive practices of care that further negate the social existence of individuals with dementia. In dementia care, social death unnecessarily precedes the physical demise of affected individuals. The concepts of habitus and symbolic violence are well suited for studying these issues in a critical yet reflexive manner. They draw attention to the complex power relations that shape medical work while interrogating the practices that destroy the self and the dignity of persons with dementia. It is imperative for an alternative discourse on decision-making to emerge, one which considers ways of seeing the person with dementia beyond the narrow parameters of measurable psychometric properties.

REFERENCES

Bamford, C. and Bruce, E. (2000) 'Defining the outcomes of community care: The perspectives of older people with dementia and their carers.' *Ageing and Society 20*, 543–570.

Beard, R.L. (2004) 'In their voices: Identity preservation and experiences of Alzheimer's disease.' *Journal of Aging Studies 18*, 415–428.

Blum, N.S. (1991) 'The management of stigma by Alzheimer family caregivers.' *Journal of Contemporary Ethnography 20*, 3, 263–284.

Bourdieu, P. (1988) *Homo Academicus*. Translated by P. Collier. Cambridge: Polity Press.

Burr, V. (1995) *An Introduction to Social Constructionism*. London: Routledge.

Chang, S.C. (1988) 'The nature of the self: A transcultural view.' *Transcultural Psychiatric Research Review 25*, 169–203.

Csordas, T. (1994) *The Sacred Self: A Cultural Phenomenology of Charismatic Healing*. Berkeley, CA: University of California Press.

Dumont, L. (1985) 'A Modified View of Our Origins: The Christian Beginnings of Modern Individualism.' In M. Carrithers, S. Collins and S. Lukes (eds) *The Category of the Person: Antropology, Philosophy, History*. Cambridge: Cambridge University Press.

Everett, J. (2002) 'Organizational research and the praxeology of Pierre Bourdieu.' *Organizational Research Methods 5*, 1, 56–80.

Fillenbaum, G.G., Landerman, L.R. and Simonsick, E.M. (1998) 'Equivalence of two screens of cognitive functioning: The Short Portable Mental Status Questionnaire and the Orientation–Memory–Concentration test.' *Journal of the American Geriatrics Society 46*, 12, 1512–1518.

Fontana, A. and Smith, R.W. (1989) 'Alzheimer's disease victims: The "unbecoming" of the self and the normalization of competence.' *Sociological Perspectives 32*, 1, 35–46.

Geertz C. (1973) *The Independence of Cultures*. New York: Basic Books.

Golander, H. and Raz, A.E. (1996) 'The mask of dementia: Images of "demented residents" in a nursing ward.' *Ageing and Society 16*, 269–285.

Gubrium, J.F. (1986) *Oldtimers and Alzheimer's: The Descriptive Organization of Senility*. Greenwich, CT: JAI Press.

Gurrera, R.J., Karel, M.J., Azar, A.R. and Moye, J. (2007) 'Agreement between instruments for rating treatment decisional capacity.' *American Journal of Geriatric Psychiatry 15*, 2, 168–173.

Harrison, C. (1993) 'Personhood, dementia and the integrity of life.' *Canadian Journal on Aging 12*, 4, 428–440.

Kim, S.Y.H., Karlawish, J.H.T. and Gurrera, R.J. (2002) 'Current state of research on decision-making competence of cognitively impaired elderly persons.' *American Journal of Geriatric Psychiatry 10*, 2, 151–165.

Kitwood, T. (1988) 'The technical, the personal, and the framing of dementia.' *Social Behaviour 3*, 161–179.

Kitwood, T. (1990) 'The dialectics of dementia: With particular reference to Alzheimer's disease.' *Ageing and Society 10*, 177–196.

Kitwood, T. and Bredin, K. (1992) 'Towards a theory of dementia care: Personhood and well-being.' *Ageing and Society 12*, 269–287.

Lai, J.M. and Karlawish, J. (2007) 'Assessing the capacity to make everyday decisions: A guide for clinicians and an agenda for future research.' *American Journal of Geriatric Psychiatry 15*, 2, 101–111.

Landrine, H. (1992) 'Clinical implications of cultural differences: The referential versus the indexical self.' *Clinical Psychology Review 12*, 401–415.

Lukes, S. (1973) *Individualism*. New York: Harper and Row.

Marson, D.C., Schmitt, F.A., Ingram, K.K. and Harrell, L.E. (1994) 'Determining the competency of Alzheimer patients to consent to treatment and research.' *Alzheimer Disease and Associated Disorders 8*, Suppl. 4, 5–18.

Matthews, E., Farrell, G. and Blackmore, A. (1996) 'Effects of an environmental manipulation emphasizing client-centred care on agitation and sleep in dementia sufferers in a nursing home.' *Journal of Advanced Nursing 24*, 3, 439–447.

Merchant, C. and Hope, K. (2004) 'The Quality of Life in Alzheimer's Disease Scale: Direct assessment of people with cognitive impairment.' *International Journal of Older People Nursing* in association with *Journal of Clinical Nursing 13*, 105–110.

Miller, B.L., Seeley, W.W., Mychack, P., Rosen, H.J., Mena, I. and Boone, K. (2001) 'Neuroanatomy of the self: Evidence from patients with frontotemporal dementia.' *Neurology 57*, 5, 817–821.

Moye, J. and Marson, D.C. (2007) 'Assessment of decision-making capacity in older adults: An emerging area of practice and research.' *Journal of Gerontology Series B: Psychological Sciences and Social Sciences 62B*, 1, P3–P11.

Orona, C.J. (1990) 'Temporality and identity loss due to Alzheimer's disease.' *Social Science and Medicine 30*, 11, 1247–1256.

Sabat, S.R. (2005) 'Capacity for decision-making in Alzheimer's disease: Selfhood, positioning and semiotic people.' *Australian and New Zealand Journal of Psychiatry 39*, 11–12, 1030–1035.

Sabat, S.R. and Harré, R. (1992) 'The construction and deconstruction of self in Alzheimer's disease.' *Ageing and Society 12*, 443–461.

Sadler, J.Z., Bernstein, B.E. and Marson, D.C. (2003) 'Legal and Ethical Aspects.' In M.F. Weiner and A.M. Lipton (eds) *The Dementias: Diagnosis, Management, and Research* (3rd edn). Washington, DC: American Psychiatric Publishing.

Sands, L.P., Ferreira, P., Stewart, A.L., Brod, M. and Yaffe, K. (2004) 'What explains differences between dementia patients' and their caregivers' ratings of patients' quality of life?' *American Journal of Geriatric Psychiatry 12*, 272–280.

Stafford, P.B. (1992) 'The nature and culture of Alzheimer's disease.' *Semiotica 92*, 1–2, 167–176.

Stewart, R. (2006) 'Mental health legislation and decision-making capacity: Autonomy in Alzheimer's disease is ignored and neglected.' *British Medical Journal 332*, 7533, 118–119.

Swartz, D. (1997) *Culture and Power: The Sociology of Pierre Bourdieu.* Chicago, IL: University of Chicago Press.

Sweeting, H. and Gilhooly, M. (1997) 'Dementia and the phenomenon of social death.' *Sociology of Health and Illness 19*, 1, 93–117.

Turner, J.H. (1991) *The Structure of Sociological Theory.* Belmont, CA: Wadsworth.

Webb, J., Schirato, T. and Danaher, G. (2002) *Understanding Pierre Bourdieu.* London: Sage.

Whitlatch, C., Feinberg, L.F. and Tucke, S.S. (2005) 'Measuring the values and preferences for everyday care of persons with cognitive impairment and their family caregivers.' *The Gerontologist 45*, 370–380.

Woods, P. and Ashley, J. (1995) 'Simulated presence therapy: Using selected memories to manage problem behaviors in Alzheimer's disease patients.' *Geriatric Nursing 16*, 9–14.

Woods, R.T. (2001) 'Discovering the person with Alzheimer's disease: Cognitive, emotional and behavioural aspects.' *Aging and Mental Health 5*, S7–S16.

CHAPTER 4

Hunting Good Will in the Wilderness

MARYLOU HARRIGAN AND GRANT GILLETT

Since the time of Immanuel Kant, the will has been regarded as a key to many questions about decision-making and rational conduct in moral philosophy. The principle of autonomy and its role in understanding medical decisions is built on the idea of a freely willed decision as an expression of rational self-government and, as such, regarded as a *sine qua non* of good clinical care. But that framework is sorely tested in the contested area of good decisions for the marginally competent, especially in care of the aged. It is often difficult to see exactly what should be recognized as a proper expression of the will of the person concerned in questionable decisions in that sphere of clinical life. We will argue that recognition of who the person is and what would be fitting in that light is the crux of such decisions. That implies that where we struggle to find an expression of will that is credible for a person wandering into the wilderness of dementia or severe cognitive impairment, we should provide what is missing out of a good will so that the cognitive wilderness does not result in an intolerable (and unethical) experience.

In the film *Good Will Hunting* (1997, Van Sant), we see a gifted young man whose abilities are not manifest until he is recognized for who he is and nurtured in the right kind of way through interaction with those who understand him. Once recognized, Will is enabled to develop his skills and show who he is but, had that not happened, he might never have expressed his true self.

What about a person with cognitive impairment? Defects in rationality may make his or her decisions look incompetent, and for that reason able to be sidelined as of no account, but we should look for ways of recognizing and evaluating those decisions with good will. We should not be blinded by our stereotype of a rational economic individual capable of his or her own decisions, but rather open to a view of persons that is less independent and more realistic in the face of understanding the frailty of the human condition. A person with cognitive impairment needs support and can no longer sustain (for self or others) the illusion of independence, but how can we develop a truly good will towards an impaired person, someone who may not fit the stereotype of a competent decision-maker?

INFLUENCES OF MODERNITY: WORLD VIEWS, IMAGES, METAPHORS

'We live in a culture that is, at least in large segments, dominated by heightened expectations of rationalism and economic productivity, so clarity of mind and productivity inevitably influence our sense of the worth of a human life' (Post 2000, p.5). In what ways do present-day world views and sociological metaphors influence the attitudes of healthcare professionals toward care of seniors and, in particular, those with dementia?

Modernity, as it emerged from the Enlightenment, provided an improved quality of life and, to a great extent, displaced the old social, political and economic hierarchies. Rationalism, with its focus on individual autonomy, resulted in 'democratic' power-knowledge locating human beings squarely in the natural world. The resulting belief in open-ended individual destiny guided by rational choice changed people's lives in Europe, North America and, indirectly, the world, and brought in its wake natural science and the Industrial Revolution. As the ideology of individualism and autonomy spread, a political framework of liberalism, the economy and the market became dominant and, through the prospect of exciting advances in science and technology, developed a stranglehold on Western thought. Among other things, that impetus resulted in rapid advances in health care but, allied with other aspects of modernity, such as bureaucratization, commercialization, commodification and corporatization, produced significant tensions in the current healthcare landscape. What is more, the person, the democratic heart of the Enlightenment, came to be seen as a 'functional' self, subject to expectations that are quite constricting (Bowie 2003; Cahoone 2003; McCarthy 1984).

Images painted by three contemporary scholars, Taylor, MacIntyre and Giddens, inform our understanding of the effect of modernism on the person. The 'looping effect of human kinds' (Hacking 1995) refers to the fact that the way we are seen comes to affect both the way we see ourselves and the way we then mould ourselves to conform to those images, effects that are deeply concerning in some situations. The first image, painted by Taylor, highlights the disengaged instrumental and individual mode of life central to modernity. Contemporary society has dissolved traditional communities and their ways of living with nature, resulting in fragmentation of identities so that those bound up in it lose their common purpose, and communities are divided. The change both removes meaning from life and 'threatens public freedom, that is, the institutions and practices of self-government' (Taylor 1989, p.500). Thus, the negative consequences are twofold: the individual experiential change devalues heroism, high purposes of life or things worth dying for; and the societal change causes disengagement and dissolution of traditional communities, marginalizing deeply entrenched values so as to replace community life with a series of mobile, changing, revocable associations (Taylor 1989; see also Taylor 1991, 1994, 2004). In such a disengaged world, where each looks after him or herself, those who are impaired inevitably fare badly.

MacIntyre (1984), another fierce critic of modernity, attacks the failure of the 'Enlightenment Project' by painting an image of 'catastrophe', all the more destructive because few are even aware of it. He argues that the unifying frameworks necessary for coherent moral discourse have been lost and fragmented so that human beings, regarded as atomistic individuals, cannot see themselves as having in common a meaning and purpose underpinning a shared conception of the ethical good. Notions of utility and of rights are disconnected fictions because one cannot argue from individual desires to an interest in the good of others or to inviolable rights for all. Enlightenment liberalism cannot therefore construct a coherent ethics able to influence institutions so that they are conducive to care and a regard for shared human excellence. Lacking any way of giving substance to that goal, institutions constantly threaten to corrupt and demoralize practitioners by subordinating the pursuit of *the Good* to that of exchangeable or marketable *goods*. Practices therefore become dominated by bureaucracies organized to gain control over lesser goods through monopoly and coercive power and equipped by those means to exploit the world as a totalizing market (MacIntyre 1984). In such a marketplace the vulnerable and powerless again lose out and become means to further the ends of others.

Giddens provides a further dramatic image, that of 'the juggernaut – a runaway engine of colossal power' which, 'collectively as human beings, we can drive to some extent but which also threatens to rush out of our control' (1990, p.139). The path of the juggernaut may be steady or erratic, but it always crushes those who try to resist it. The ride may bring certain rewards in that it may be exhilarating and charged with hopeful anticipation; however, because it escapes reflective guidance, its effects are uncertain. The journey is uncontrolled and the terrain burdened with risks so that ambivalent feelings of ontological security and existential anxiety are generated. Four dialectically related frameworks of experience intersect in significant ways: estrangement and familiarity; intimacy and impersonality; expertise and reappropriation; and abstract systems and day-to-day knowledgeability. Thus, the imagery of the juggernaut of modernity is not an engine with integrated machinery, but rather one that includes multiple, often contradictory, influences (Giddens 1990). Its power and impetus, however, leave no time to reflect and consider the value of that which is fragile and elusive.

Two principal kinds of institutions in our society, the market and bureaucracy, are powerful steering mechanisms that operate in impersonal ways, remove moral responsibility for decisions that are made, and dominate health care. Together they give rise to decisions that are, 'in a sense, in their aggregate form decided by nobody' (Taylor 1994, p.175), and as a result constantly threaten to corrupt practices. A permeating ethos then develops with an emphasis on efficiency that incorporates and insulates efficient managers who characteristically attempt to affect the actions of others (by manipulation rather than by rational argument) but, in thrall to a corporate agenda, do not respond to anyone who lacks power particularly if they challenge valorized outcomes (MacIntyre 1984).

Hughes (2001, p.86) contends that '[t]he conceptual view we have of the person will affect the care we are prone to give' to those with severe dementia. Malloy and Hadjistavropoulos (2004) argue that a person's ontological position informs the perception of the self and others and defines the groundwork for all human interaction, including how caregivers and managers perceive patients and those they manage:

> The 'science' of management, bureaucracy and institutionalism is based on the premise that individuals are defined by their roles within the health care facility; people fulfil their designated obligations and must accept a loss of personal freedom in exchange for wages and security and the assurance that the 'system' runs well. (p.150)

No concern needs to be expressed for the meaning that the worker takes from his or her job or the ontological nature of the relationship among staff and patients. Within this framework, organizational efficiency requires objective (rather than inter-personal) relationships between caregivers and patients (Kitwood and Bredin 1992).

Stein (2001), in discussing the cult of efficiency, claims that, as the language of efficiency or cost-effectiveness infiltrates the public institutions of health care and education, physicians, nurses and teachers are expected to work under that ethos as an end in itself and adopt it as a value more important than others. Consequently, when efficiency is elevated to an end rather than a means, the discussions obscure the individuals involved and their individual value. Saul (1999) observes that efficiency does not produce direction and that management is not leadership – it does not provide meaning, ideas or purpose but rather 'works effectively as a function or servant of policy' (p.11). There is, he contends, a growing dependency on managers who focus on efficiency at the expense of genuine effectiveness, a tendency that produces an increase in passivity and frustration among doctors, nurses and other health professionals who resent 'being locked up in corporations'. As a mere functionary, he says, one cannot influence policy or choose directions of development, even when information is available from those who work in the system and appreciate its internal dynamics.

In these ways 'world view and metaphor become intertwined and develop into reflections of each other' (Post 2000, p.33), so our metaphors and analogies must be scrutinized, because they define our interpretation of the world and of people with dementia. Managerialism sees the world as packages or processes that deliver commodities, and 'a good that becomes a commodity is also fundamentally redescribed...it is valued in a different way...its instrumental value becomes highlighted, rather than whatever intrinsic value it may have previously been thought to possess' (Hanson 1999, p.268). The moral significance of personhood and self-understanding is a casualty of seeing persons with impaired cognition as mere consumers to be satisfied. As such, their intrinsic worth as individuals is necessarily eclipsed by more general measures.

THE IMMEASURABILITY OF PERSONS

Emmanuel Levinas, deeply shaken by the events of the holocaust in which human beings were herded like cattle (albeit efficiently and with maximum efficacy) into places that treated them as numbers of documentable (and ultimately disposable) items, explored the idea that a person is an enigma replete with value, who challenges us morally beyond all our stereotypes (Levinas 1996). He prompts us to notice that each human being is an irreplaceable colloquy of skills and traces of the past living amongst us, addressing us, making implicit demands for engagement and recognition. Every human individual is multiply inscribed by the experiences of a life journey that no one else will ever take, and carries with them things of value that once lost can never be recovered. We are called to recognize these life stories and witness them in ways that are fitting. Depending on their impairments, vulnerabilities and dependencies, we can seek ways of helping the individuals involved to enact those stories in new contexts and in the face of challenges they did not choose to confront.

> It is paradoxical that an epoch which has exalted individualism virtually to the supreme value should have had so gross a disregard for individuality. Behind the ideology it was, of course, merely an economic individualism that was espoused. The truth is that each of us has our own history, personality, likes, dislikes, abilities, interests, beliefs, values and commitments, and our unique identity is made up through some combination of these (Kitwood 1994, p.11).

Modernity has inherited the ideology that a person is a conscious self-determining individual and that to be a person is to have certain criterial psychological properties. The human individual, seen thus, is a joint product of self-directed choices and a physical substrate – the body. States of the self are states of that psychosomatic individual; and as a person, the individual makes choices which demand legal and economic respect. When a human being no longer fits this mould, he or she is regarded as impaired, and a strange disconnect occurs whereby the rights the person enjoys diminish to the right to life, relief of suffering (in so far as that is possible) and physical integrity.

By contrast, a more realistic notion of a situated and intrinsically relational self stresses context and the complex factors that contribute to a person's being-in-the-midst-of-others. Each of us is a node of personal and discursive activity and influences which energize and validate a person so that his or her story is filled with life and with meaning. Taylor asserts that a basic condition of making sense of ourselves is 'that we grasp our lives in a narrative' (1989, p.34). Such narratives are created in community against horizons of meaning where events stand out as personally and collectively important and the involvement of each person with others who care enhances both the personal and shared meanings of the events concerned.

MacIntyre (1984) contends that there is no way of *founding* one's identity – or lack of it – on the psychological continuity or discontinuity of the self as an isolated person making individual choices which are equalized or 'flattened' (to borrow Taylor's term): 'The self inhabits a character whose unity is given as the unity of character [of an individual in a given socio-cultural context]' (MacIntyre 1984, p.217). Once again, modernity and hyper-individualism do not provide what the narrative concept of selfhood requires: that I am what I may properly be taken by others to be in the course of living out a story that runs from my birth to my death. I am the subject of a history that is my own and no one else's; it has its own peculiar meaning and, within that story, I am accountable for the actions and experiences which compose a liveable (and creditable) life.

In what does the unity of an individual life consist? The answer is that its unity is the unity of a narrative embodied in a single life. To ask 'What is the good for me?' is to ask how best I might live out the unity and bring it to completion. To ask 'What is the good for man?' is to ask what all answers to the former question must have in common. The unity of a human life is the unity of a narrative quest (MacIntyre 1984).

These thoughts explain why we might say 'Sometimes an individual needs a story more than food to stay alive' (Lopez 1990, p.60). That story is not merely an individual creation, although in it an individual is created (and in part self-created) as a being-in-relation-to-others. Buber (1959) frames one way of relating to another as I–It, and a second way as I–Thou. A relationship in the I–It mode implies information-gathering, objectivity, instrumentality – engagement without commitment. Relating in the I–Thou mode, however, requires involvement – a risking of ourselves and a moving towards. Frank (2004) describes a 'generosity' that is required by relations of dialogue, of face-to-face encounters, and makes them more than mere informational exchanges. Such discourse is not merely speech; it is an encounter in which we add reality and depth to each other's configured narratives. We do this, or should do it, with good will, a will that has a sense of life and sees the narrative for what it is, that recognizes persons as persons. 'Ultimately, the narrative has ethical content because it impacts on the body and what the body must endure' (Gillett 2004, p.26). In health care the bodies of professionals are also involved, carrying with them the inscriptions of the past and affecting the ways that the professional acts.

In exploring frameworks of personhood one must therefore ask whether the rationality of modernist individualism is too severe a ground for moral standing. The isolated individual evaluated as a being complete in him or herself is a fiction but, dangerously, an alienated fiction like 'a fish out of water', gasping for narrative and personal life. The metaphors should alert us to the scaffolding with which we all live and that supports us (keeps us from falling over), and gives purchase to our cognitive skills. The moral context of care may frame issues surrounding care in alignment with rationality or by using other ways of understanding personhood. Both Levinas (1996) and Nelson (2001) allow us to speak of individuals being acknowledged, treated as sacred and held in being as what MacIntyre (1999) calls 'dependent rational individuals'.

Each of us is constantly a being-in-the-process-of-becoming who has to adapt to the world in new ways; and one is not alone in this task but is held in personhood by relationships which support us and enhance our abilities. In the film *Away From Her* (2007, Polley), we see Fiona adapting to the changes of her dementia, supported by Aubrey, her new companion in the nursing home. Her husband learns a new way of supporting her, recognizing that she needs Aubrey to be a part of her evolving life.

Where does this leave the debate, currently centred on critical and experiential reasons, about decision-making in states of impaired cognition? Does it not suggest that something more informal and caring, some reasons accepting the many indeterminacies and the non-self-contained or rationally integrated nature of human identity, should inform us?

DECISION-MAKING FOR PERSONS IN THE WILDERNESS: IMPLICATIONS FOR THE CAREGIVER

The capacity to value is a reflection of being a person situated in a life context with horizons of meaning. Jaworska (1999) argues that the ability to value is independent of the ability to understand the narrative of one's whole life, and that people with dementia may well retain the former ability long after they lose the latter. She may be right, but that focus tends to narrow our focus to the psychological individuals adrift in the experiential wilderness of dementia, whereas central to one's personhood is the capacity to espouse values and convictions rooted in a meaningful context and to translate them into action (with assistance) in ways that, for the person concerned, represent a good will. Dworkin (1993), to some extent, recognizes this fact when he argues that the central point is capacity for autonomy, and that it should translate into a respect for critical interests as the most authentic interests of the person concerned. But this does not mean that we should focus exclusively on wishes or expressed preferences whether present (experiential) or critical.

MacIntyre affirms the significance of virtue, practice and community. Virtues are valued as inherent moral goods because they enable the individual and society to live well and can be understood as dispositions that sustain practice and enable one to achieve the goods internal to practice. They also sustain a quest for the good by increasing self-knowledge and increasing knowledge of the good as conceived and aimed at in communities in which members seek the good together (MacIntyre 1981). The integrity of a practice therefore depends on the way in which the virtues are encouraged in sustaining institutions that support that practice because it 'requires the exercise of the virtues by at least some of the individuals who embody it in their activities' (MacIntyre 1984, p.195). Decisions for those in the wilderness can only be made in the presence of virtues commensurable with one's own (shared) conception of the good.

Decision-making reflecting one's own character, values, commitments, convictions and (both critical and experiential) interests is not the same as being in charge of one's life presently or precedently, but is rather the experience of living according to the dictates of a good will – a will aligned with one's own good as seen in the light of a responsive appreciation of who one is. In essence, this is a regard for patient dignity – the preciousness and fragility of the good that is realized in a given person. Professionals who recognize that are what one wishes for as companions on the path of care when one has strayed into the wilderness. Those in the wilderness still need a 'place to stand' (however unsteady they may be when unaided) – a need that requires of the professional an understanding of the complexities, moral sensibilities, values and present joys of the individual concerned, all of which must be weighted with phronesis (or practical wisdom) informed by a sense of life (Gillett 2004).

To safeguard patient dignity, the 'connecting, synthesizing link is the morality of civic equality' but this is not mere equality of flattened economic or experiential wishes, rather an ethic of inter-personal civility and consideration. This can only be nested in a broad framework of understanding, embracing profession–society and professional–patient relations situated in the space of common citizenship (Sullivan 1999, p.11), where individuals are valued and recognized as irreplaceable members of the organic reality that is our shared being-in-the-world-with-others. When that is a lively feature of our interactions with the cognitively impaired, suitably informed by a sense of life – a sense that life is an adventure, and that part of its joy precisely is the confrontation with the new (Nussbaum 1990) – we move to a type of care that is itself enlivening and affirming, so that a partnership emerges in which a detached assessment of critical or experiential interests is not to the point. Engagement and the appreciation of narrative identity together suggest a different way of caring focused on the individual as an individual and not merely as a consumer of a care package, generated and costed to meet the rational requirements of a modernist conception of the human self-serving individual.

REFERENCES

Bowie, A. (2003) *Introduction to German Philosophy: From Kant to Habermas*. Cambridge: Polity Press.
Buber, M. (1959) *I and Thou*. Edinburgh: T. and T. Clark.

Cahoone, L. (ed.) (2003) *From Modernism to Postmodernism: An Anthology* (2nd edn). Malden, MA: Blackwell.

Dworkin, R. (1993) *Life's Dominion: An Argument about Abortion, Euthanasia, and Individual Freedom.* Toronto: Random House.

Frank, A.W. (2004) *The Renewal of Generosity.* Chicago, IL: University of Chicago Press.

Giddens, A. (1990) *The Consequences of Modernity.* Stanford, CA: Stanford University Press.

Gillett, G.R. (2004) *Bioethics in the Clinic: Hippocratic Reflections.* Baltimore, MD: Johns Hopkins University Press.

Hacking, I. (1995) *Rewriting the Soul: Multiple Personality and the Sciences of Memory.* Princeton, NJ: Princeton University Press.

Hanson, M.J. (1999) 'Biotechnology and commodification within health care.' *Journal of Medicine and Philosophy 24,* 3, 267–287.

Hughes, J.C. (2001) 'Views of the person with dementia.' *Journal of Medical Ethics 27,* 2, 86–91.

Jaworska, A. (1999) 'Respecting the margins of agency: Alzheimer's patients and the capacity to value.' *Philosophy and Public Affairs 28,* 105–138.

Kitwood, T.M. (1994) 'The concept of personhood and its implications for the care of those who have dementia.' *Care-Giving in Dementia: Vol. 2.* London: Routledge.

Kitwood, T. and Bredin, K. (1992) 'Towards a theory of dementia care: Personhood and well-being.' *Ageing and Society 12,* 269–287.

Levinas, E. (1996) *Basic Philosophical Writings.* Bloomington, IN: Indiana University Press.

Lopez, B. (1990) *Crow and Weasel.* Toronto: Random House.

MacIntyre, A. (1981) *After Virtue: A Study in Moral Theory.* London: Gerald Duckworth.

MacIntyre, A. (1984) *After Virtue: A Study in Moral Theory* (2nd edn). Notre Dame, IN: University of Notre Dame Press.

MacIntyre, A. (1999) *Dependent Rational Animals: Why Human Beings Need the Virtues.* Chicago and LaSalle, IL: Open Court.

Malloy, D.C. and Hadjistavropoulos, T. (2004) 'The problem of pain management among persons with dementia, personhood, and the ontology of relationships.' *Nursing Philosophy 5,* 147–159.

McCarthy, T. (1984) 'Translator's Introduction.' In J. Habermas (T. McCarthy, trans.) *The Theory of Communicative Action: Vol. 1. Reason and the Rationalization of Society.* Boston, MA: Beacon Press.

Nelson, H.L. (2001) *Damaged Identities, Narrative Repair.* Ithaca, NY: Cornell University Press.

Nussbaum, M.L. (1990) *Love's Knowledge: Essays on Philosophy and Literature.* New York: Oxford University Press.

Post, S.G. (2000) *The Moral Challenge of Alzheimer Disease: Ethical Issues from Diagnosis to Dying* (2nd edn). Baltimore, MD: Johns Hopkins University Press.

Saul, J.R. (1999) 'Health Care at the End of the Twentieth Century: Confusing Symptoms for Systems.' In M.A. Somerville (ed.) *Do We Care? Renewing Canada's Commitment to Health: Proceedings of the First Directions for Canadian Health Care Conference.* Montreal: McGill-Queen's University Press.

Stein, J.G. (2001) *The Cult of Efficiency.* Toronto: House of Anansi Press.

Sullivan, W.M. (1999) 'What is left of professionalism after managed care?' *Hastings Center Report 29,* 2, 7–13.

Taylor, C. (1989) *The Sources of Self.* Cambridge, MA: Harvard University Press.

Taylor, C. (1991) *The Malaise of Modernity.* Toronto: House of Anansi Press.

Taylor, C. (1994) 'Philosophical Reflections on Caring Practices.' In S.S. Phillips and P. Benner (eds) *The Crisis of Care: Affirming and Restoring Caring Practices in the Helping Professions.* Washington, DC: Georgetown University Press.

Taylor, C. (2004) *Modern Social Imaginaries.* Durham, NC: Duke University Press.

CHAPTER 5

A Confucian
Two-Dimensional Approach
to Personhood, Dementia,
and Decision-Making

DANIEL FU-CHANG TSAI

Healthcare professionals charged with the care of dementia patients are constantly faced with an ethical dilemma: for patients with dementia so advanced that identity, personality, and preferences have changed to the point that he or she has seemingly become another person, whose wishes or choices in terms of medical care or life and death decision should healthcare professionals choose to respect and follow? Should it be the earlier, pre-dementia person's wishes or the later, post-dementia onset person's preference?

A common solution to such an ethical dilemma is to follow established guidelines concerning medical decision-making for incompetent patients. The order for making such decisions in the United States, according to long-established court rulings, is commonly: first, advance directives or advance care planning with patients; second, the surrogate's decision based on patients' preferences; and third, the doctor's judgment of the best interest for the patients (Lo 2000). However, dementia patients are not always incompetent, and when they possess a changed identity, personality, or personhood, the above decision-making flow chart may not be applicable, and the dilemma is still to be resolved. One general rule for resolving such an ethical dilemma is that the surrogate decision-maker or the healthcare team should at this time consider the long-lasting, stable identity, personality, or personhood that has been established across the lifetime of the person with dementia, and decide which choice is most compatible with or preferred by such identity, personality, or personhood, since it is the autonomy of this person that we seek to respect.

An even more challenging, but nonetheless common, ethical question is: Should persons with dementia receive aggressive treatments such as endotracheal intubation with respirator, hemodialysis for renal failure, cardiac pulmonary resuscitation (CPR), or even extra-corporeal membrane oxygenation (ECMO) for the purpose of prolonging life? Among these common yet tough clinical choices lies the fundamental ethical question: If persons with dementia have lost orientation, memory, thought, consciousness, and rationality permanently, do they still possess the same "person" or "moral" status—that is, the "moral personhood"—as other people and therefore deserve the same respect including full medical care? In other words, an important philosophical question to answer is: What is the "personhood" of dementia patients and how will this influence medical decision-making?

THE TRADITIONAL CONCEPTION OF PERSONS

Conceptions of personhood have been complex and diverse, leading to deep controversies in Western philosophy in general, and modern bioethics in particular. Traditional thinking presupposes all human beings—the species *Homo sapiens*—to be persons as an indisputable, self-evident truth. Devine (1987) described this as the "species principle"; human organisms are persons no matter their degree of maturity or decay, whereas non-human animals, robots, or extraterrestrial life cannot be persons. Since the Judeo-Christian traditions see human beings as having been created in the image of God, and human dignity and rights flowing from God's creation, they also assert that all human beings are persons. However, these traditionalist conceptions of personhood are challenged by bioethical dilemmas. Should an embryo or fetus, without any likeness to human beings, share the same dignity and rights as persons? Should someone with advanced dementia or in a permanent vegetative state still be treated as a "person"?

MODERN BIOETHICAL CONCEPTIONS OF PERSON: THE CAPACITY CRITERIA

Many philosophers and bioethicists from a liberal point of view argued against the traditional position and separated "persons" from "human beings." That is, if a "human being" were not at the same time a "person," he would have no human rights because, as Engelhardt (1986) suggests, "Persons, not humans, are special" (p.104). Nevertheless, how is "person" defined? In modern Western philosophy, Descartes defined "person" as a "thinking thing." John Locke (1964) was the first to distinguish "person" from "human being"; it was his view that the latter only means a corporeal existence, whereas the former is "a thinking intelligent being that has reason and reflection and can consider itself, the same thinking thing, in different times and places" (p.286). Most importantly, according to Kant, to be a person is to be a rational agent capable of exercising freedom as autonomy. Thus, all of these traditional philosophers differentiate between a person and a human being, drawing attention to the role of thinking rationally as the defining criterion.

In modern bioethics, this trend to distinguish between a human being and a person continues. Singer (1979) distinguished two meanings of human beings: one, a member of the species *Homo sapiens*; two, a being possessing certain qualities which, based on Fletcher's (1972) proposed list for "indicators of humanhood," are self-awareness, self-control, a sense of the future, a sense of the past, the capacity to relate to others, concern for others, communication, and curiosity. Singer defined that only human beings in the second sense are "persons" who deserve rights and respect and, furthermore, that the crucial characteristics of persons are rationality and self-consciousness. Warren (cited in Rudman 1997) similarly distinguished a "genetic sense" and a "moral sense" of being human. She confined personhood to the moral sense by giving five criteria including: consciousness and in particular the capacity to feel pain; reasoning; self-motivated activity; the capacity to communicate messages of an indefinite variety of types; and the presence of self-concepts and self-awareness. According to her, the first feature alone (consciousness and the capacity to feel pain) could constitute personhood. Tooley (1987) also indicated that a person must have the awareness of self as a continuing entity and be capable of having an interest in his own continued existence. Harris (1985) argued that a person is "any being capable of valuing its own existence" (p.18). Engelhardt (1986) proposed that a general secular moral community presumes a community of entities who are self-conscious, rational, free to choose, and in possession of a sense of moral concern. He defined those who had these four characteristics as *persons strictly*. On the other hand, human beings such as infants, those with profound intellectual impairment, the permanently comatose, and individuals suffering from advanced Alzheimer's disease, who lack those characteristics, are merely *social persons*—that is, they are persons just for social considerations.

Although these various conceptions have different emphases on what should be counted as the standards of personhood, they all stress that *rationality, self-consciousness,* and *autonomous moral agency* are the key features of persons. In effect, the bioethical principle of respect for autonomy is largely established on this foundation that persons are rational, self-conscious, autonomous moral agents who have liberty and the right to choose for themselves, and should therefore be treated with the utmost respect. This perspective has traditionally grounded Western approaches to bioethics and understanding of personhood. Eastern philosophies would seem to counter this perspective.

THE CONFUCIAN TWO-DIMENSIONAL APPROACH TO PERSONS

Confucius is one of the most influential thinkers of Eastern philosophy and could be seen as a representative of Eastern culture. Among the world's great philosophers, Confucius is regarded as one of four paradigmatic individuals (together with Socrates, Gautama Buddha, and Jesus Christ), owing to the extended influence through two millennia and the extraordinary importance for all philosophy that each has had (Jaspers 1962).

Within Confucian philosophy, like the Judeo-Christian traditional conception, there is no philosophical distinction between "human being" and "person." Furthermore, there is only one word, *jen*, in the Chinese language to stand for the Western terms "human being" (*Homo sapiens*) and "person." It was only during the last few decades that a new term *wei-ger* was coined to translate and introduce the concept of "personhood" into academic discourse. Nevertheless, Confucian philosophy has its particular theories and conceptions of persons which, one could argue, implicitly address notions of personhood.

Mencius' and Hsun Tzu's emphases on persons

Mencius, who is generally considered to be the greatest successor of Confucius, said: "*Slight is the difference between men and the brutes.* The common man loses this distinguishing feature, while the superior man (*chun-tze*) retains it..." (Lau 1984, p.165, italics added). It is the ability to feel that appears to distinguish man from brute. As Mencius argued:

When I say all men have the mind which cannot bear to see the suffering of others, my meaning may be illustrated thus: Now, when men suddenly see a child about to fall into a well, they all have a feeling of alarm and distress, not to gain friendship with the child's parents, nor to seek the praise of their neighbours and friends, nor because they dislike the reputation [of lack of humanity if they did not rescue the child]. From such a case, we see that a man without the feeling of commiseration is not a man; a man without the feeling of shame and dislike is not a man; a man without the feeling of deference and compliance is not a man; and a man without the feeling of right and wrong is not a man. The feeling of commiseration is the beginning of humanity [sic: humaneness] (jen); the feeling of shame and dislike is the beginning of righteousness (yi); the feeling of deference and compliance is the beginning of propriety (li); and the feeling of right and wrong is the beginning of wisdom (zhi). Men have these Four Beginnings just as they have their four limbs. Having these Four Beginnings, but saying that they cannot develop them, is to destroy themselves... If anyone with these Four Beginnings in him knows how to give them the fullest extension and development, the result will be like fire beginning to burn or a spring beginning to shoot forth. When they are fully developed, they will be sufficient to protect all people within the four seas. (Chan 1969, pp.65–66)

According to Mencius, then, what distinguishes men from animals are the inborn moral capacities of humaneness (jen), righteousness (yi), propriety (li), and wisdom (zhi). He calls these the Four Beginnings. These moral potentialities bring worth and dignity to one's life and make persons worthy of respect, yet these Four Beginnings need to be realized. Obviously, the natural moral capacity of feeling right or wrong is a faculty of rationality, whereas the feelings of commiseration, shame and dislike, and deference and compliance require the agent to be a self-reflective person. From this point of view, Mencius' definition of person is not incompatible with the modern Western conceptions of personhood. However, it is unclear whether human beings who cannot develop (e.g., severely intellectually delayed infants) or who have lost such capacities (the advanced Alzheimer or permanently comatose patients)—thereby in Mencius' terms possessing, in essence, no moral faculties of humaneness, righteousness, propriety, and wisdom—can still be counted as persons by Mencius.

Hsun Tze, another prominent successor of Confucius, argued differently. He begins to shift the focus from the individual to a social being:

Men do not have the strength of bulls, nor do they run as fast as horses, yet why are bulls and horses mastered by men? All because men are capable of social organisation while animals are not. (Cited in Hui 2000, p.104; author's translation)

He emphasized an important perspective of persons—the relational dimension. His work begins to highlight how, in the Confucian traditions, a person is always conceived of as a part of a network of relations rather than an isolated, individual entity. From this perspective, what distinguishes human beings from animals is, first, the natural endowment of men's potential capacity to achieve *jen* (humaneness) and *yi* (righteousness) and, second, the "human sociality." This explains why Mencius said, "The compass and the square produce perfect circles and squares. By the sage, human relations are perfectly exhibited" (Legge 1991b, p.292; translation modified by author).

Confucius' conception of persons

Confucius' conception of persons has been interpreted through his moral ideal of a *chun-tze* (the superior man) and has encapsulated two dimensions—the vertical dimension (the autonomous, self-cultivating one) and the horizontal dimension (the relational, altruistic one) (Tsai 2001). This two-dimensional approach sees a person not only as a rational, autonomous agent but also as a relational, altruistic identity whose self-actualization involves incessant participating in and promoting of the welfare of his fellow persons. *Chun-tze* in Confucius' ethics is the man of high moral achievement who constantly tries to improve and cultivate himself to attain various stages of perfection. Many characteristics of a *chun-tze* reflect the two-dimensional approach thoroughly.

The concept of *chun-tze* comprises various meanings that are commensurate with the idea of autonomous persons, reflecting the vertical dimension of Confucian personhood. According to the Confucian Classics, this morally ideal person (*chun-tze*) possesses the characteristics of self-activation (Legge 1963), self-cultivation (Chan 1969), self-reflection (Legge 1991b), self-reliance (Legge 1991a), and moral authenticity (Chan 1969; Legge 1991a). Actually, the superior man is well qualified to be an autonomous person, a true moral agent, since he sees himself as the master of his own life and attributes all responsibilities to himself and not to someone else. He is a self-starter and self-legislator; he refuses to be controlled or coerced by others and unceasingly searches and cultivates in himself the virtues of humaneness. The goal of Confucius' moral philosophy and moral education in reality is to create an autonomous person who is self-activated, self-determined, self-reliant, and is constantly improving himself via moral self-cultivation.

However, apart from being an autonomous person, *chun-tze* has another prominent feature as emphasized in Confucius' ethics, that is, the relational perspectives. The central theme of Confucius' ethics, "humaneness" (*jen*), which in the Chinese character means two persons and is pronounced in the same way as the Chinese word "human," reflects the idea of relational personhood because the Chinese concept of man is based on *"the individual's transactions with his fellow human beings" (Hsu 1971, p.29, italics in original)*. "Ethics"'in Confucian philosophy in particular and daily life in general simply refers to the ideal interpersonal relationships, as the author defines it—the horizontal dimension of being persons. Thus, in the Confucian sense:

> [M]an is not an ultimately autonomous being who has an inner and decisive power, intrinsic to him, a power to select among real alternatives and thereby to shape a life for himself. Instead he is born as "raw material" who must be civilized by education and thus become a truly human being. (Fingarette 1972, p.34)

Echoing this understanding, Liang Shu-ming identified that "In the Chinese thinking, individuals are never recognised as separate entities; they are always regarded as part of a network, each with specific role in relation to others" (cited in Tao 1996, p.11). He proposed that the traditional Chinese is neither individual-based nor society-based, but relational-based (cited in King and Bond 1985). Tu Wei-ming also pointed out that "self" in the classical Confucian sense is both "a centre of relationships" and "a dynamic process of spiritual development" (Tu 1985, p.113). He suggests that "one becomes fully human through continuous interaction with other human beings and that one's dignity as a person depends as much on communal participation as on one's own sense of self-respect" (p.55). In other words, a Confucian person is socially situated, defined, and shaped in a relational context where he must achieve humaneness (*jen*) through interaction with other particular individuals. No one can be fully human without playing roles in the interaction with one's fellow persons. Put differently:

> [T]he self develops its contours, unfolds its characteristics, takes shape, becomes actual and individuated through engaging and interacting in a network of relations with others... Self-individuation is possible only through a process of engagement with others within the context of one's social roles and relationships. (Tao 1996, p.16)

Apart from stressing the relatedness rather than separateness of personhood, the Confucian selfhood also needs to be mentioned for relevance in two ways.

First, the boundaries between self and others are not always clear in Chinese philosophy. The self, as the center of relations, is not merely "a privatised self, the small self and a self that is a closed system" (Tu 1985, p.58). Instead, it can be and should be broadened to become a public-spirited, great self and a self that is an open system (Tu 1985) that deepens in self-transformation through genuine communication with others. Family, community, country, and the world, from the Confucian point of view, are spheres of selfhood where one engages in promoting them and transforming oneself. As Elvin indicated:

> Perhaps this absence of alienation from the world gave the self in China slightly less sharply defined margins than it had in the West. For the Chinese, this life was neither a vale of tears, nor a testing-ground, but a home. (Cited in Tao 1990, p.123)

Second, the Confucian self searches in unity with *dao*. In Chinese philosophy, *dao* symbolizes the universal moral order and the ideal status of moral achievement for man to define, pursue, and accomplish. Metaphysically, man realizes his *true self*, the "true manhood" when he lives in unity and harmony with *dao*. Put differently, the universal moral order is a purpose that invites and demands the participation of man; man is likewise inspired by the *dao* in his ceaseless pursuit and transformation to be in unity with *dao* (Legge 1963). Therefore, the self in Confucius' ethics is not alienated from the universe. The true self, in its sincere pursuit of *dao*, participates and thus transforms the universe as well. This is beautifully explicated in *Chung-yung* (*The Doctrine of the Mean*):

> Only those who are absolutely sincere can fully develop their nature. If they can fully develop their nature, they can then fully develop the nature of others. If they can fully develop the nature of others, they can then fully develop the nature of things. If they can fully develop the nature of things, they can then assist in the transforming and nourishing process of Heaven and Earth. If they can assist in the transforming and nourishing process of Heaven and Earth, they can thus form a trinity with Heaven and Earth. (Chan 1969, pp.107–108)

In summary, the ideal Confucian person, *chun-tze*, not only fulfills the requirement of an autonomous person but also is a man of virtues and commitments towards family and society. He pursues harmonious relationships with man and *dao*, and is featured with two major components that are mutually dependent—moral self-cultivation (the vertical dimension) and altruism towards others (the horizontal dimension). For Confucianism, rationality is historically and culturally grounded; "well-tested social practices and tradition provide sound...foundations for meaningful life" (Lee 1994, p.50). When a *chun-tze* exercises his autonomy rationally and self-consciously, he is not choosing in a context-free manner but locating himself in a certain moral-historical tradition. The cardinal concern and meaning of life for the Confucian person lies in fulfilling his duties in the various roles he plays, creating and maintaining the harmonious relationships with people and nature, contributing to the flourishing of human society, and ultimately being at one with the *dao*. The conception of persons is thus shifted from emphasizing the *individual* to the *individual's relationships plus an other-regarding morality with altruistic responsibility*. Therefore, the Confucian sense of human dignity and worth places more emphasis on a moral accomplishment for one to attain, and less on a given fact of capacity that one is born with.

In contrast, the Western modern (bioethical) conception of persons emphasizes that they are autonomous, rational, and self-conscious individuals who are "making context-free choice in a conceptual vacuum" (Lee 1994, p.50) and are capable of identifying and pursuing their own good. Being conceived of as sovereign agents of choices, persons hence deserve equal concern and respect for the inviolability of their rights and privacy; *even collective goals and good are not sufficient reasons to compromise them*. In other words, it is a person's separateness, individuality, and distinctiveness rather than his relatedness, mutuality, and communion with others that are valued. To sum up this general contrast between Chinese and the West using Hansen's description, "Western theorists have understood the world as made up of particulars. Chinese metaphysical theory analyses objects as parts carved out of a large, more basic whole" (Hansen 1997, p.108).

CONCLUSION

Dementia causes persons to lose their mental, verbal, communicative, and social capacities, at first gradually and then more profoundly. According to the capacity criteria of modern bioethical personhood, when dementia patients lack the capacity of self-awareness, self-control, a sense of the future, a sense of the past, the capacity to relate to others, concern for others, communication, and curiosity (to use Fletcher's criteria) or simply rationality, self-consciousness, and autonomous moral agency, they no longer possess a moral personhood. In Engelhardt's (1986) terms, advanced dementia patients, who are devoid of the four characteristics of being self-conscious, rational, free to choose, and in possession of a sense of moral concern, are merely persons in the social sense, not persons in the strict sense. Bluntly, from this viewpoint, dementia patients in the advanced stages are only "human beings" but not "persons" anymore and, therefore, health care provided to them could be—or even should be—less than that given to patients with full capacity of personhood. Consequently, withholding, withdrawing, or terminating treatments or life support from them should arouse little or no ethical controversy at all, since they are no longer "persons" of moral significance.

Yet, this is clearly contradictory to most people's common moral intuition as well as to existing general social or medical practice. Modern bioethical criteria for personhood as applied to dementia patient care seem problematic.

In contrast, based on the Confucian conception of personhood, dementia patients may have lost their capacity for rationality, self-consciousness, and autonomous moral agency for ever, which means, in Mencius' terms, losing the moral faculties of humaneness, righteousness, propriety, and wisdom—the Four Beginnings of being persons. They may therefore lack the characteristics of the vertical (autonomous) dimension of being persons. However, they still possibly possess the characteristics of the horizontal (relational) dimension of being persons. This could be understood in two senses. First, persons with dementia have, through genuine communion with and altruistic efforts towards other fellow persons in their lifetime, achieved the horizontal (relational) dimension of persons; human dignity and worth is a moral accomplishment they have earned. Second, no matter what degree of decay or degeneration dementia disease has caused the patients, the relatedness, connectedness, and dependence among them and their families, friends, and fellow persons will most likely remain existent; this most fundamental human love and affection cannot be denied by theories that define personhood in terms of capacity criteria. This love and affection of mutual relatedness and interconnectedness usually continues to mean something (or even a great deal) for the families and friends of the dementia patients, even if it is not equally felt by the patients themselves owing to advancement of disease symptoms. This means that the personhood of the dementia patient has never been entirely lost because this horizontal, relational dimension of persons is not gone in them.

For these reasons, the healthcare needs and medical rights of dementia persons continue to deserve our prudent consideration. Even if dementia patients do not always receive the extensive and full range of medical intervention, they are still due basic, decent healthcare and life support. Withholding or withdrawing aggressive or advanced medical treatment for them cannot be based on the rationale that they are no longer persons. It must be because such treatments are not in their best interest. Deciding what is in the best interest for dementia patients is never easy, especially in the context of health care. The values, wishes and preferences of dementia patients expressed before their dementia are by all means a central and decisive consideration, since this is based on the principle of respect for autonomy which mandates that we show our respect for the still-persons. However, according to the above arguments, the relational, horizontal dimension of personhood should also play an important role, especially when its importance has increased after people have developed dementia. In other words, in addition to the prior expressed values and preferences of persons with dementia, the relationship of love and affection between these persons and their families and friends should have a role in helping to decide what is in their best interest.

In conclusion, according to the Confucian two-dimensional approach, the diminishment and elimination of rationality, consciousness, and autonomous agency caused by dementia will deprive the individual of the vertical (autonomous) dimension of personhood from persons, but it cannot take away the horizontal (relational) dimension of personhood since this has been realized through interpersonal transactions over their lifetime, and it remains recognized and regarded by their fellow persons. Such dimension and relation will still be valued by those related to persons with dementia, continue to play a certain role, and be taken into consideration in decision-making for the health care of the dementia patient. The Confucian two-dimensional approach to personhood when applied to dementia patient care is more ethically plausible and hence socially acceptable.

ACKNOWLEDGMENT

This chapter is developed from the author's earlier works and particularly from:

Tsai, D.F. (2001) "How should doctors approach patients? A Confucian reflection on personhood." *Journal of Medical Ethics 27*, 1, 44–50.

The author wants to thank the National Research Program for Genomic Medicine (NRPGM) of the National Science Council of Taiwan for supporting this research.

REFERENCES

Chan, W.T. (1969) *A Source Book in Chinese Philosophy.* Princeton, NJ: Princeton University Press.

Devine, P.E. (1987) "The Species Principle and the Potential Principle." In B. Brody and H.T. Engelhardt (eds) *Bioethics: Readings and Cases.* Englewood Cliffs, NJ: Prentice-Hall.

Engelhardt, H.T. (1986) *The Foundations of Bioethics.* New York: Oxford University Press.

Fingarette, H. (1972) *Confucius: The Secular as Sacred.* New York: Harper and Row.

Fletcher, J. (1972) "Indicators of humanhood: A tentative profile of man." *The Hastings Center Report 2*, 5, 1–4.

Hansen, C. (1997) "Chinese Philosophy and Human Rights: An Application of Comparative Ethics." In G.K. Becker (ed.) *Ethics in Business and Society: Chinese and Western Perspectives.* Hong Kong: Springer.

Harris, J. (1985) *The Value of Life.* London: Routledge.

Hsu, F.L.K. (1971) "Psychological homeostasis and jen: Conceptual tools for advancing psychological anthropology." *American Anthropologist 73*, 23–44.

Hui, E. (2000) "Jen and Perichoresis: The Confucian and Christian Bases of the Relational Persons." In G.K. Becker (ed.) *The Moral Status of Persons: Perspectives on Bioethics.* Amsterdam and Atlanta, GA: Rodopi.

Jaspers, K. (1962) *The Great Philosophers.* London: Rupert Hart-Davis.

King, A.Y.C. and Bond, M.H. (1985) "The Confucian Paradigm of Man: A Sociological View." In W.S. Tseng and D.Y.H. Wu (eds) *Chinese Culture and Mental Health.* Orlando, FL: Academic Press.

Lau, D.C. (trans) (1984) *Mencius.* Hong Kong: Chinese University Press.

Lee, K.S. (1994) "Some Confucianist reflections on the concept of autonomous individual." *Journal of Chinese Philosophy 21*, 49–59.

Legge, J. (trans) (1963) *The I Ching.* New York: Dover Publications.

Legge, J. (trans) (1991a) *Confucian Analect: The Chinese Classics. Vol. I.* Taipei: SMC Publishing.

Legge, J. (trans) (1991b) *Mencius: The Chinese Classics. Vol. II.* Taipei: SMC Publishing.

Lo, B. (2000) *Resolving Ethical Dilemmas: A Guide for Clinicians* (2nd edn). Philadelphia: Lippincott Williams & Wilkinson.

Locke, J. (1964) *An Essay Concerning Human Understanding: Book II.* London: Oxford University Press.

Rudman, S. (1997) *Concepts of Person and Christian Ethics.* Cambridge: Cambridge University Press.

Singer, P. (1979) *Practical Ethics.* Cambridge: Cambridge University Press.

Tao, J. (1990) "'The Chinese moral ethos and the concept of individual rights." *Journal of Applied Philosophy 7*, 2, 119–127.

Tao, J. (1996) "The Moral Foundation of Welfare in Chinese Society: Between Virtues and Rights." In G.K. Becker (ed.) *Ethics in Business and Society: Chinese and Western Perspectives.* Hong Kong: Springer.

Tooley, M. (1987) "The Criterion of Awareness of Self as a Continuing Entity." In B. Brody and T.H. Engelhardt (eds) *Bioethics: Reading and Cases.* Englewood Cliffs, NJ: Prentice-Hall.

Tsai, D.F.C. (2001) "How should doctors approach patients? A Confucian reflection on personhood." *Journal of Medical Ethics 27*, 1, 44–50.

Tu, W.M. (1985) *Confucian Thought: Selfhood as Creative Transformation.* New York: State University of New York Press.

CHAPTER 6

Cultural Safety, Decision-Making and Dementia
Troubling Notions of Autonomy and Personhood[1]

WENDY HULKO AND LOUISE STERN

Interactions between service providers and the recipients of services, such as older persons with dementia, have been the focus of concerted efforts to ameliorate the effects of difference – to achieve the goal of 'working across difference' (Narayan 1988). Power features prominently in all of these relationships, particularly when there is a difference in cognitive capacity and age that places the service provider in an advantaged position in relation to the service user. Markers of cultural difference – the norms, values, beliefs, traditions and practices that signal membership in a particular social group – subtly shape our day-to-day actions and profoundly influence interactions between the providers and the recipients of services in dementia care, as in any other health or social service encounter. 'Culture' is one of the many lenses through which we see and make sense of the world; and recognizing cultures as 'taking on meanings through webs of narratives' (Dhamoon 2006, p.359) highlights the socially constructed and context-contingent nature of culture.

While much has been written about culture and dementia, in particular how culture mediates our understandings of dementia and use of services (see Mackenzie, Bartlett and Downs 2005), several thorny issues have yet to be fully addressed, let alone resolved. One particular issue is the potential conflict between person-centred care or a personhood focus (specific to dementia care) on the one hand and a culturally appropriate or culturally safe approach (general to health and social care) on the other. A central question is: how might a person-centred approach take into consideration cultures that do not value the individual over the collective and that do not see autonomy as the gold standard? In an attempt to address this question, we introduce the concept of 'cultural safety', developed in 1990 by Irihapeti Ramsden (2005), and apply it to two cases that showcase different yet comparable aspects of this problematic: a First Nations female elder with memory loss living at home on her reserve and an older Jewish man with dementia living out his last days in a Jewish care facility. The work that follows is largely theoretical and conceptual, so as to set the stage for the empirical chapters that follow. It builds on concerns with the limitations of personhood approaches (see Hulko 2002) and arises from a shared focus on 'hearing the voice[s] of people with dementia' (Goldsmith 1996) and placing dementia in a socio-cultural context (Downs 2000). It is these two traditions (personhood and context) that we are trying to reconcile; in doing so, we have chosen to trouble the concepts of autonomy and personhood, which are strongly valued – and understandably so – within dementia care.

This chapter starts with an introduction to cultural safety, followed by a brief review of the theoretical concepts of autonomy and personhood and an overview of the limitations of autonomy-based approaches to decision-making. This is followed by a description of two cases that highlight and suggest tensions that can occur in practice with respect to preserving personhood and respecting culture, and our analysis of these cases with respect to cultural safety. The chapter concludes with suggestions as to how to move forward in practice and research in order to preserve personhood *and* respect culture, without essentializing the latter or isolating the former.

THE CULTURAL AND CULTURAL SAFETY

This work embraces Dhamoon's (2006) shift away from 'culture' towards 'the cultural': culture is a problematic concept, largely due to the frequency with which it is conflated with ethnicity and race (see Desflor Edles 2004; Oommen 1994) and the tendency to treat it as static and immutable; in other words, culture is 'tainted by essentialism', while the cultural 'focuses on socially trans-mitted knowledge and behaviour which is not homogeneously taken to have the same meaning for all people' (Dhamoon 2006, p.10). Similarly, cultural safety focuses on the fluidity of culture and the power relations that mark all cross-cultural interactions, in contrast to culturally aware, culturally sensitive and culturally competent approaches to care that ignore power and often take a tick-box (essentialist) approach to culture (Johnstone and Kanitsaki 2007; NAHO 2008; Wepa 2005). Dianne Wepa (2007) stresses that while becoming culturally aware (seeing oneself as having culture and noticing difference) is an important first step, it is really 'a shift in power' from the service provider to the service recipient that distinguishes cultural safety from cultural sensitivity.

Cultural safety is closely tied to indigenous peoples' struggles towards self-determination and decolonization and has been referred to as critical social theory (NAHO 2006) due to its focus on power relations and transformational agenda. Like personhood, cultural safety is a desired outcome of an approach to care that seeks to change power relations: the care associated with the former concept is focused on improving relationships between people who are cognitively impaired and those who are cognitively well, while the relation-ships of primary importance for cultural safety are those between the colonizer and the colonized. 'Developed by non-dominant Maori peoples reacting to negative experiences in the health and nursing system' (NAHO 2006, p.1), cultural safety seeks to value that which is often devalued, namely the voices and experiences of minoritized people.

> Cultural safety requires that health care providers be respectful of nation-ality, culture, age, sex, political and religious beliefs, and sexual orienta-tion. This notion is in contrast to transcultural or multicultural health care, which encourages providers to deliver service irrespective of these aspects of a patient. Cultural safety involves recognizing the health care provider as bringing his or her own culture and attitudes to the relationship. (NAHO 2008, p.4)

Although first articulated by indigenous peoples to apply to interactions between Maori (colonized) and Pakeha (colonizer), cultural safety has been adopted as a model of care that can and should be used with all cultural groups who share a marginalized position in relation to the White Anglo-Canadian norm (NAHO 2006, 2008; see also Wepa 2005). There is also a recognition within this model that people do not belong to only one cultural group, that other aspects of their identities such as their gender expression, age and sexual orientation are equally salient. This is important to take into account when con-sidering decision-making and dementia, as, for example, people who are in same-sex relationships face the challenge of ensuring recognition of their partner or a member of their 'chosen family' as their substitute decision-maker largely due to heteronormativity and homophobia (Haley *et al.* 2002; O'Connor, Phinney and Hulko forthcoming 2010).

PERSONHOOD AND AUTONOMY

Personhood-oriented approaches to dementia and person-centred care arose from the seminal work of Tom Kitwood and his colleagues at the University of Bradford (see Baldwin and Capstick 2007; Kitwood 1997). The 'standard paradigm' (Kitwood 1988) of dementia with its bio-medical orientation and prescriptions, and the 'malignant social psychology' (Kitwood 1990) surrounding people with dementia, were found to depersonalize persons with dementia, through tactics such as infantilization, labelling, outpacing and banishment (Kitwood 1990). Thus, Kitwood advocated for concerted efforts to acknowledge and maintain the 'personhood' of individuals living with dementia, as this 'standing or status that is bestowed upon one human being, by others, in the context of relationship and social well-being' (1997, p.8) is not always afforded people with dementia. Rather, personhood – as something that we all should have by virtue of being humans – is taken for granted until we develop dementia and all our actions and decisions become circumspect. The ability of dementia to compromise an individual's autonomy rests on the acceptance of a worldview that values autonomy above all else. This worldview predominates in healthcare ethics and medical decision-making and features prominently in the codes of ethics for several professions, including social work, the profession to which both authors belong.

> Social work is founded on a long standing commitment to respect the inherent dignity and individual worth of all persons. When required by law to override a client's wishes, social workers take care to use the minimum coercion required. Social workers recognize and respect the diversity of Canadian society, taking into account the breadth of differences that exist among individuals, families, groups and community. (CASW 2005)

Individuals in need of health care are treated as autonomous beings from whom healthcare practitioners are required to seek informed consent; and this consent may only be gained from another legally recognized party (a substitute decision-maker) if the individual in need of care has demonstrated a lack of capacity to give informed consent on their own behalf. The primacy of the individual is unquestioned within this ethical-legal decision-making framework.

When dementia is implicitly equated with incapacity, family members or next of kin, who are not necessarily legal 'substitute decision-makers', may be asked to sign proxy consent forms, without anyone assessing the person with dementia's capacity to consent or ascertaining their views on the proposed treatment or research, for example. In an attempt to make the consent process more meaningful for, and inclusive of, persons with dementia, researchers have chosen to make use of ongoing negotiated or process consent (Allan 2001; Dewing 2002, 2007; Hubbard, Downs and Tester 2003; Reid, Ryan and Enderby 2001). This method of gaining informed consent/assent arises from a commitment to personhood and a concern with ensuring the voice and inclusion of persons with dementia regardless of their degree of impairment. Such efforts, which involve ascertaining the degree to which persons with dementia assent (if their consent cannot be obtained or is not considered legally valid), and then continuing to negotiate this throughout the research process, undoubtedly rest on notions of autonomy and concern with promoting the rights of the individual. Ongoing negotiated consent is certainly an improvement over traditional informed consent protocols for both research and practice. However, do personhood-focused approaches such as these implicitly reinforce culturally bound beliefs about autonomy and individualism; and if so, can/should this be justified? This question has led us to look more closely at concerns with autonomy-based approaches to decision-making and to interrogate these concerns in relation to the people with whom we work as researchers and practitioners.

CONCERNS WITH AUTONOMY-BASED APPROACHES TO DECISION-MAKING

The notion of the autonomous decision-maker (whose opinion we need to solicit and decisions we need to abide by, so long as they are capable) guides much of the contemporary practice and research in the field of dementia, particularly interventions stemming from a person-centred approach. This occurs in spite of the cultural relativity (non-universality) that clearly marks such Western, individualistic conceptions of decision-making and advance care planning (Bowman and Singer 2001; Kwak and Haley 2005; Searight and Gafford 2005; Seymour *et al.* 2004; Widdershoven and Berghams 2001). Many cultural groups view decision-making as a collective, rather than an individual (autonomous), activity and for this reason, among others, decision-support tools such as advance directives or living wills are not well used, nor is the appointment of a single substitute decision-maker necessarily favoured (see

Haley *et al.* 2002; Kwak and Haley 2005). The *process* of advance care planning is generally thought to be more culturally appropriate (culturally safe) than decision-making *tools* such as advance directives (see Widdershoven and Berghams 2001). Culturally safe decision-making necessitates the meaningful involvement of the service recipient in the decision-making process, the provision of specific explanations for recommended courses of action, and respect for the need to consult with family before making a decision (NAHO 2008; see also Chapleski, Sobeck and Fisher 2003). Autonomy-based decision-making likely would not be a culturally safe way of working with either First Nations or Jewish persons.

DECISION-MAKING AND DEMENTIA IN FIRST NATIONS CULTURE

There has been very little research on dementia and First Nations older adults (Cammer 2006; Henderson and Henderson 2002; Hulko 2007), despite this being acknowledged as a gap in the literature in the few research studies undertaken over a decade ago (Hagan Hennessy and John 1996; Hendrie *et al.* 1993; John *et al.* 1996; Pollitt 1997). While dementia has been observed in older people in almost all populations, some researchers feel that this is 'basically a Western diagnostic category' (Pollitt 1996, p.2). At the same time, healthcare providers believe that dementia is 'under-recognized and under-addressed in Northern and aboriginal populations' (Cammer 2006, p.13; see also Jervis and Manson 2007). As to First Nations' decision-making processes and roles in the context of dementia, little information can be gleaned from the few studies to date on dementia and indigenous peoples. What has been identified as important is the holistic perspective on health and well-being (Pollitt 1997; see also Reading, Kmetic and Gideon 2007), particularly the spiritual aspect, with a few researchers having discovered that symptoms of dementia are viewed as communication with the other side and can facilitate a closer connection with one's ancestors or the spirit realm (Henderson and Henderson 2002; Henderson and Traphagan 2005; O'Connor *et al.* forthcoming 2010). Ensuring the inclusion of aboriginal older adults with memory loss in decision-making requires viewing them as embedded within a collective, retaining a focus on the community as a whole, and attending to their physical, spiritual, mental and emotional health and well-being.

Collective decision-making is more the norm than is autonomous decision-making in First Nations communities (Chapleski *et al.* 2003; Hagan Hennessy and John 1996; Parrack and Joseph 2007) where the health and well-being of each and every individual is a collective responsibility and an indicator of the survival and healing of the community (Lafontaine 2006; Reading *et al.* 2007). The entire band may be involved in decision-making with respect to an individual member, as it is recognized that all members have a role to play in determining and upholding the collective decision and that no one is simply 'a person' – we are all embedded within families and communities, and these relationships that shape and nurture us are far more important than a sense of autonomy (Hart 2002; NAHO 2008). As elder Mike Arnouse[2] explained:

> First Nations cultures are generous and caring and help one another and take care of the Earth. Everything is related. Dementia is rather new among our Native nations now because of our culture being destroyed – our language, 'cause that's where the stories come from, our language mainly. There are few people that still remember some of the culture and the ways of life of our people that have been passed down from time immemorial. We're getting less and less of elders – so it's a matter of time for us to gather this information before it's totally destroyed. I guess dementia has a lot to do with destruction of a people's way of passing history on – the truth, you know. So the relationship between the colonizer and the colonized changed into…something that we can do or work together to change our attitudes to contribute recognition to the ones who still hang onto their culture. And the ones I mean that hang onto their culture are the original people of this Turtle Island.[3] Because we have contributed a lot to the world already and if the relationship between the colonizer and the colonized becomes better we both can contribute towards making it a better place to leave for our future generations and all the other living beings that share this land with us – the feathered ones and the four-legged, the ones that live in the water, the tiny little creatures, the medicines. (Personal communication, 17 January 2008)

These cultural values and this collective approach to decision-making are exemplified in the following description of a female First Nations elder with memory loss. The woman in this case study is not identified or labelled as having dementia, as this is not a term that is used in First Nations communities and this phenomenon is not viewed as particularly problematic either. Memory loss is not the defining characteristic of her life. Her status as an elder, not simply an older person (see Stiegelbauer 1996), is far more important, particularly with respect to decision-making.

Alice – A First Nations elder living
at home on the reserve

Alice is one of the oldest living persons on her rural reserve in British Columbia and a well-respected elder in her community. Now in her eighties, she lives with a son who has dedicated his life to taking care of her, although her daughter also lives on the reserve, as do several of her other sons. Both the family and the community view Alice as 'the boss' – she is the one they gather around and to whom they listen. Each year on her birthday, the whole community comes together to celebrate and some of the other elders tell stories of her life. This helps her and everybody else to retain their memories of history. Alice has short-term memory loss: she has trouble remembering names and stories of the recent past, yet remembers stories from long ago. She does not like to speak about residential school[4] and all that is related to this (i.e. compensation payments, residential school survivor support) because the memories are 'not good' – not because she does not remember what happened to her and to her schoolmates. Alice's repetitions of stories and use of humour helps everyone in her community to learn lessons from the past and that humour is one of the great medicines for survival and healing. A home support worker visits Alice weekly, and on Friday afternoons workers from a day program in the local town pick her up and take her to play cards, then give her a bath and cut her nails. When decisions need to be made about Alice and her care, the entire family is involved and decisions are based on family and community, with Alice being central to this. If she doesn't want to go to hospital, she won't go and the family will honour her decision, unless she is really sick, in which case the family will make a decision to take her so that she can get the care they can't provide. The family advises support workers who ask them how to work with Alice: 'Visit with her, don't just ask questions, she'll tell stories – serious stories, funny stories. The stories she tells are ones she's heard from others. If you see cards on the table, play cards with her and then maybe she'll let you do the dishes. If there's wood outside, chop some of it for her. The most important thing is not to be too clinical or mechanical. This will open up friendship and respect and she'll begin to speak more freely.'

This story is about an older woman with memory loss who is entwined with her family and community. She is clearly not an autonomous decision-maker; however, this does not appear to be due to her memory loss per se, rather it is consistent with the cultural as expressed in her community. Decisions are made collectively, and she is the one to whom others look for guidance. In collectivist cultures, a sense of self is more embedded in the community than in the individual (Waid and Frazier 2003); that Alice is still very much a person to those who surround her and is not experiencing 'a loss of self' is therefore not altogether surprising.

A worldview such as this, which assigns value to a person in the context of who they are, rather than what they can do, also underlies Jewish bio-ethics and decision-making with respect to persons with dementia, as is evident in the next section on decision-making within a Jewish cultural context that precedes our second case study. This next case study looks at a different point along the continuum of dementia, to the end-of-life, in order to further demonstrate how alternative conceptualizations of autonomy and decision-making are problematized and experienced through a cultural lens.

DECISION-MAKING WITHIN A JEWISH CULTURAL CONTEXT

In Jewish culture, the principles of Jewish law (Halacha) have provided a guiding ethical framework for decision-making in the context of medical treatment and intervention. These laws are derived from the foundational texts of the Bible and the Torah and guide not just religious practices and beliefs, but a variety of aspects of everyday life. From the perspective of medical ethics and decision-making, the following principles are foundational:

- the sanctity and preservation of life are paramount
- the quality and duration of life is irrelevant
- the notion of unlimited personal autonomy is rejected
- humans are 'called beings' with duties and obligations in addition to rights.

A key point to the Jewish medical ethics approach to individuals with dementia, especially as they near the end-of-life, is the inherent belief that they 'retain their human dignity and are as worthy of protection as those who are healthy' (Jotkowitz, Clarfield and Glick 2005, p.881). Therefore, all inter-personal behaviour in Judaism is traditionally conceived as the execution of duties within the context of relationships (Goldsand, Rosenberg and Gordon

2001) and often in the context of filial duty, obligation and responsibilities, rather than as 'rights' (Jotkowitz *et al.* 2005).

In this framework, the concept of individual autonomy is voluntarily limited in that it must be kept consistent with Jewish law (Kinzbrunner 2004). Thus, individuals or families directly consult with their rabbis to ensure that they have correctly interpreted Jewish law as it relates to specific decisions regarding medical treatment and care, for example. Within the Jewish community, there exists a myriad of interpretive views on issues pertinent to dementia care, specifically as they relate to the treatment options at the end-of-life (Gillick 2001). It is important to note that it is impossible to capture and represent a unanimous Jewish voice due to the heterogeneous and diverse nature of Judaism, and there have been critiques raised that traditional Jewish bio-medical ethics based on textual precedents are not in sync with the speed and complexity of modern-day medicine and technology, or the diverse nature of Jewish identity itself (Solomon 2001). However, according to Goldsand *et al.* (2001), Jewish bio-ethics is a framework that can be embraced by all Jews regardless of their adherence and affiliation with the faith:

> To traditionally minded Jews, Jewish bioethics is a subset of Halacha. To more secular Jews, seeking guidance in difficult decisions about their health, Jewish bioethics offers helpful lessons and considered opinions from the sages. Many non-religious Jews welcome traditional views to help ease the uncertainty inherent in difficult decisions, even though they may not live according to traditional religious practice. (p.220)

The emphasis on decision-making is centred therefore on the valuing of an individual's life in the context of themselves as individual incarnation of G–d,[5] as family member, as community member and as a Jew. The individual is not seen as a separate entity devoid of context, but as an interdependent piece of a larger puzzle. This becomes problematic when it butts up against the liberal rights-based medical ethics that dominates health care and that tends to favour autonomy of the individual. In fact, current ethical thinking in medicine does not tend to conform to the religious and cultural norms of specific groups, Jewish people and First Nations people being two clear examples.

It is also important to note that in examining decision-making within a Jewish context as it applies to people with dementia, we cannot ignore the ethno-historical context of this generation of Jewish elders and their families. This is a generation raised with the spectre of anti-Semitism, the war, the Holocaust and forced emigration. Therefore, it comes as no surprise that experiences of aging, ill health and death and dying are often skewed to the experiences of the past. Care within a Jewish environment may be sensitive to the needs of this group, but upon entry into the mainstream medical system, an adherence to culturally specific frameworks of decision-making becomes problematic and often the demarcator of 'difference'.

The following case study illustrates the ways in which individual or personal autonomy is precluded by 'duty' and the ethno-historical factors of oppression and resistance; and how these decisions are questioned and analysed using a different and opposing framework – a unique cultural lens.

Edward – An older Jewish man living in a Jewish care facility

Edward was a 76-year-old Jewish man in the end stages of Alzheimer's disease residing in a Jewish long-term care facility. The progression of the disease had resulted in his inability to eat safely, and it took the staff an inordinate amount of time to feed him. He was constantly aspirating and developing pneumonia, which led him to multiple hospital admissions. Both Edward and his brother Herman had been imprisoned during the war in a concentration camp and they were the only two surviving members of their family. At Herman's insistence, Edward remained a 'full code' for medical intervention. Very few of the facility's residents were 'full codes' due to the intrusive and invasive nature of such interventions for individuals who were already compromised. While Edward had rejected Judaism after he was liberated from the camp, Herman remained religious and consulted his rabbi on most matters. With Edward's continuing decline and constant re-hospitalizations, Herman demanded a gastric feeding tube for Edward. Herman stated that, as an observant Jew, it was his right to demand that Edward continue to be treated at the highest level of intervention. Only G–d had the power to take a life. Edward was not suffering, but he would be if he were not nourished properly. Herman became irate with the healthcare team when they questioned the validity of this choice because the tube would not keep Edward alive, and would be intrusive and painful. Herman accused the care team of trying to kill Edward and threatened to take legal action if the tube was not inserted. The inter-disciplinary team was made up of individuals from a myriad of ethno- and socio-cultural groups, including Jewish. Many people on the team felt torn between their understanding of and empathy with Edward's and Herman's past and their connection to one another, versus their belief that prolonging Edward's life was cruel and unnatural. All the team members felt that Edward should be left to let nature take its course. In rounds and case review, many team members felt that it was because the brothers were Jewish that Herman could not accept Edward's impending death. This oft-spoken belief had become a truism to the team and was rarely challenged because of the fact that any previous experiences with families 'in denial' were with Jewish families, not surprisingly because that is who constituted the client base.

BALANCING CULTURAL SAFETY AND PERSONHOOD

The histories of Jewish people and of First Nations people are marked by horrific attempts to eliminate not only the culture and way of life of these two distinct groups, but also their very beings – through the pogroms in Eastern Europe, the invasion and colonization of Turtle Island, the Holocaust and residential schools to contemporary expressions of anti-Semitism and racism. Understandably, both First Nations people and Jewish people prefer to 'care for their own' and may be distrustful of healthcare providers who do not share their cultural background. In turn, this affects how they approach decision-making and the concept of autonomy. A practitioner striving to ensure cultural safety for Alice and Edward would be aware of his/her own social location, particularly his/her ethno-cultural ancestry, and would recognize the history of harms enacted on the cultural groups to which Alice and Edward belong and that they have experienced in their individual lives as members of historically disadvantaged groups. The service provider would work to effect the requisite shift in power, which requires a non-clinical approach (playing cards) with Alice and a quite technical approach (putting in a feeding tube) with Edward. The intervention would be considered culturally safe if those on the receiving end deemed it so.

Following a culturally safe decision-making model would require fully involving the family (however this may be defined by Alice and Edward) and deferring to their decision-making authority if this is consistent with the wishes of Alice and Edward. This becomes problematic in the end stages of dementia, when an individual's ability to express his/her wishes is precluded by his/her inability to communicate using conventional methods, and healthcare providers cede decision-making powers to family members (substitute decision-makers) in reaction to these losses. In the case of Edward, for example, the decisions made on his behalf by his brother were not necessarily in keeping with his individual wishes, but they did fulfil a greater need to exert control and challenge the medical culture's conceptualization of how a person should die, irrespective of dementia diagnosis. Within other cultures, decision-making is primarily seen to be the duty of the family as a form of obligation and protection, regardless of an individual's cognitive status (Chan 2004; Kagawa-Singer and Blackhall 2001), and this is evident in both of these cases which reflect two ends of the illness trajectory.

In promoting cultural safety, we are cautious of the need to ensure that the person with dementia is not lost in the process (i.e. that 'the cultural card' is not used to justify preventing the person with dementia from being involved in decision-making or ignoring their clearly expressed wishes). Yet, as demonstrated above, this is often difficult as it becomes so tangled up with past histories and oppressions, which can play out quite dramatically on people who have lived with this legacy. The effects of this legacy can be quite different as well, depending on degree of acculturation (see Chapleski *et al.* 2003) and proximity to past atrocities like residential schools and the Holocaust. As the cultural is flexible and context-contingent and interacts with other identity factors such as age and gender, we should not assume that all older people will hold the same expectations and desires with respect to family involvement and care planning.

CONCLUSIONS

Unevenly balanced with our concerns about the appropriateness of an 'autonomy-based approach to decision-making' is the issue of who has the power to define concepts such as decision-making, informed consent and capacity in the context of dementia. This critique of power relations within dementia care is more consistent with a person-centred approach as it hints at a desire for greater involvement of people with dementia and recognition of their voices as individuals. It also recognizes that people with dementia reside within a network of relationships and contexts that have the power to shape their experiences. To date, people with dementia have not had any definitional power by virtue of their diminished capacity. The definition of culture we put forth at the outset, along with the idea that the cultural is socially constructed, could enable us to view people with dementia as a cultural group, one with a shared meaning-making system and identity. This is not an attempt to homogenize people with dementia or to conceal differences within this cultural group in terms of other signifiers of identity, like ethnicity, gender, race, class, age, sexual orientation, faith and (dis)ability. Rather, it opens space for questions like: (1) What kind of approach to decision-making might be favoured by people with dementia as a cultural group, and should we reject an autonomy-based approach to decision-making?; (2) How might allegiance to other cultural groups formed around additional identity categories such as ethnicity and 'race' shape the views of people with dementia on decision-making and personhood?; and (3) How do we respond to the increasing prevalence of cross-cultural care in the communities and institutions that people with dementia inhabit, and how should that affect dementia care? Addressing questions such as these could assist efforts to place persons with dementia in the centre in terms of decision-making without losing sight of the circles that surround and support them. This balancing act is necessary for those concerned with focusing not only on individuals, but also on families, communities and institutions, none of which are uniform or homogeneous.

ACKNOWLEDGEMENTS

We would like to acknowledge Mike Arnouse, an elder from Adams Lake Indian Band, and all the First Nations people who have shared their knowledge in the spirit of healing mistakes made in the past and creating better relationships between aboriginal and non-aboriginal peoples.

ENDNOTES

1. We are using the idea of 'trouble' in two ways in this chapter – to indicate that we are making problematic these 'normative' concepts in the tradition of Judith Butler (see Butler 1999), and that these concepts may be of concern with or without our efforts to trouble them.

2. Mike Arnouse is an elder adviser to the first author's First Nations' Perspective on Dementia research project and offered these words of wisdom specifically for the purpose of inclusion in this book chapter.

3. Turtle Island is the name the original inhabitants of North America gave to this continent.

4. Approximately 130 residential schools operated in Canada from the 1800s to the 1980s, with the majority being run by the Catholic Church (Indian Residential School Survivors Society, n.d.). Aboriginal children were forcibly removed from their homes and communities in a historical event that has been termed 'cultural genocide' (Jack 2006). Children aged 7–15 years were beaten for speaking their native language and interacting with their siblings, regularly endured psychological and emotional abuse, and were subjected to severe physical and sexual violence (Indian Residential School Survivors Society, n.d.; Jack 2006. Up to 60 per cent of the students died (Indian Residential School Survivors Society, n.d.)), and those who survived continue

to struggle with the impact of this horrific experience, as do their children and grandchildren (Smith, Varcoe and Edwards 2005). On 11 June 2008 the Prime Minister of Canada, Stephen Harper, made a statement of apology to former students and 'sought forgiveness for the students' suffering' (Office of the Prime Minister 2008).

5. Out of respect for the conservative and orthodox Jewish traditions, the authors have similarly chosen to reference that faith's higher power without directly writing the name.

REFERENCES

Allan, K. (2001) *Communication and Consultation: Exploring Ways for Staff to Involve People with Dementia in Developing Services.* Bristol: The Policy Press.

Baldwin, C. and Capstick, A. (eds) (2007) *Tom Kitwood on Dementia: A Reader and Critical Commentary.* Maidenhead: Open University Press.

Bowman, K. and Singer, P. (2001) 'Chinese seniors' perspectives on end-of-life decisions.' *Social Science and Medicine 53,* 455–464.

Butler, J. (1999) *Gender Trouble: Feminism and the Subversion of Identity.* New York: Routledge.

Cammer, A.L. (2006) 'Negotiating culturally incongruent healthcare systems: The process of accessing dementia care in Northern Saskatchewan.' Unpublished master's thesis, University of Saskatchewan, Saskatoon, Canada.

Canadian Association of Social Workers (CASW) (2005) *Code of Ethics.* Retrieved 14 November 2008 from www.casw-acts.ca.

Chan, H.M. (2004) 'Sharing death and dying: Advance directives, autonomy and the family.' *Bioethics 18,* 2, 87–103.

Chapleski, E.E., Sobeck, J. and Fisher, C. (2003) 'Long-term care preferences and attitudes amongst Great Lakes American Indian families: Cultural context matters.' *Care Management Journals 4,* 2, 94–100.

Desflor Edles, L. (2004) 'Rethinking "race", "ethnicity" and "culture": Is Hawai'i the "model minority" state?' *Ethnic and Racial Studies 27,* 1, 37–68.

Dewing, J. (2002) 'From ritual to relationship: A person-centred approach to consent in qualitative research with older people who have a dementia.' *Dementia 1,* 2, 157–171.

Dewing, J. (2007) 'Participatory research: A method for process consent with persons who have dementia.' *Dementia 6,* 1, 11–25.

Dhamoon, R. (2006) 'Shifting from "culture" to "the cultural": Critical theorising of identity/difference politics.' *Constellations 13,* 3, 354–373.

Downs, M. (2000) 'Dementia in a socio-cultural context: An idea whose time has come.' *Ageing and Society 20,* 369–375.

Gillick, M.R. (2001) 'Artificial nutrition and hydration in the patient with advanced dementia: Is withholding treatment compatible with traditional Judaism?' *Journal of Medical Ethics 27,* 12–15.

Goldsand, G., Rosenberg, Z.R.S. and Gordon, M. (2001) 'Bioethics for clinicians: 22. Jewish bioethics.' *Canadian Medical Association Journal 164,* 2, 219–222.

Goldsmith, M. (1996) *Hearing the Voice of People with Dementia: Opportunities and Obstacles.* London: Jessica Kingsley Publishers.

Hagan Hennessy, C. and John, R. (1996) 'American Indian family caregivers' perceptions of burden and needed support services.' *Journal of Applied Gerontology 15*, 3, 275–293.

Haley, W.E., Allen, R.S., Reynolds, S., Chen, H., Burton, A. and Gallagher-Thompson, D. (2002) 'Family issues in end-of-life decision-making and end-of-life care.' *American Behavioral Scientist 46*, 2, 284–298.

Hart, M.A. (2002) *Seeking Mino-Pimatisiwin: An Aboriginal Approach to Helping.* Halifax, NS: Fernwood.

Henderson, J.N. and Henderson, L.C. (2002) 'Cultural construction of disease: A "supernormal" construct of dementia in an American Indian tribe.' *Journal of Cross Cultural Gerontology 17*, 197–212.

Henderson, J.N. and Traphagan, J.W. (2005) 'Cultural factors in dementia: Perspectives from the anthropology of aging.' *Alzheimier's Disease and Associated Disorders 9*, 4, 272–274.

Hendrie, H., Hall, K., Pillay, N., Rodgers, D. *et al.* (1993) 'Alzheimer's disease is rare in Cree.' *International Psychogeriatrics 5*, 1, 5–14.

Hubbard, G., Downs, M. and Tester, S. (2003) 'Including people with dementia in research: Challenges and strategies.' *Aging and Mental Health 7*, 5, 351–362.

Hulko, W. (2002) 'Making the Links: Social Theories, Experiences of People with Dementia and Intersectionality.' In A. Leibing and L. Scheinkman (eds) *The Diversity of Alzheimer's Disease: Different Approaches and Contexts.* Rio de Janeiro: CUCA-IPUB.

Hulko, W. (2007) 'Exploring First Nations' perspectives on dementia.' Retrieved 14 November 2008 from www.interiorhealth.ca/uploadedFiles/Health_Services/Aboriginal_Health/TRU.pdf.

Indian Residential School Survivors Society (n.d.) 'History' Retrieved 4 January 2009 from www.irsss.ca/history.html.

Jack, A. (ed.) (2006) *Behind Closed Doors: Stories from the Kamloops Indian Residential School.* Penticton, BC: Theytus Books.

Jervis, L.L. and Manson, S.M. (2007) 'Cognitive impairment, psychiatric disorders, and problematic behaviours in a tribal nursing home.' *Journal of Aging and Health 19*, 2, 260–274.

John, R., Hagan Hennessy, C., Roy, L.C. and Salvini, M.L. (1996) 'Caring for Cognitively Impaired American Indian Elders: Difficult Situations, Few Options.' In G. Yeo and D. Gallagher-Thompson (eds) *Ethnicity and the Dementias.* Washington, DC: Taylor and Francis.

Johnstone, M. and Kanitsaki, O. (2007) 'An exploration of the notion and nature of the construct of cultural safety and its applicability to the Australian health care context.' *Journal of Transcultural Nursing 18*, 3, 247–256.

Jotkowitz, A.B., Clarfield, A.M. and Glick, S. (2005) 'The care of patients with dementia: A modern Jewish ethical approach.' *Journal of the American Geriatric Society 53*, 5, 881–884.

Kagawa-Singer, M. and Blackhall, L.J. (2001) 'Negotiating cross-cultural issues at the end-of-life: "You gotta go where he lives."' *Journal of the American Medical Association 286*, 23, 2993–3001.

Kinzbrunner, B.M. (2004) 'Jewish medical ethics and end-of-life care.' *Journal of Palliative Medicine 7*, 4, 558–566.

Kitwood, T. (1988) 'The technical, the personal, and the framing of dementia.' *Social Behaviour 3*, 2, 161–179.

Kitwood, T. (1990) 'The dialectics of dementia: With particular reference to Alzheimer's disease.' *Ageing and Society 10*, 2, 177–196.

Kitwood, T. (1997) *Dementia Reconsidered: The Person Comes First.* Buckingham: Open University Press.

Kwak, J. and Haley, W.E. (2005) 'Current research findings on end-of-life decision-making among racially or ethnically diverse groups.' *The Gerontologist 45*, 634–641.

Lafontaine, C. (2006, 27 November) 'Presentation to the Senate Standing Committee on Aging.' Retrieved 14 November 2008 from www.naho.ca/publications/ agingPresentation.pdf.

Mackenzie, J., Bartlett, R. and Downs, M. (2005) 'Moving towards culturally competent dementia care: Have we been barking up the wrong tree?' *Reviews in Clinical Gerontology 14*, 1–8.

Narayan, U. (1988) 'Working together across differences: Some considerations on emotions and political practice.' *Hypatia 3*, 2, 31–47.

National Aboriginal Health Organization (NAHO) (2006) 'Fact sheet: Cultural safety.' Retrieved 14 November 2008 from www.naho.ca/english/documents/Culturalsafetyfactsheet.pdf.

National Aboriginal Health Organization (NAHO) (2008) *Cultural Competency and Safety: A Guide for Health Care Administrators, Providers and Educators.* Ottawa, ON: National Aboriginal Health Organization.

O'Connor, D., Phinney, A. and Hulko, W. (forthcoming 2010) 'Dementia at the intersections: A unique case study exploring social location.' *Journal of Aging Studies 24*, 1.

Office of the Prime Minister (2008, 11 June) 'PM offers full apology on behalf of Canadians for the Indian Residential Schools system.' Retrieved 4 January 2009 from www.pm.gc.ca/eng/media.asp?category=1&id=2146.

Oommen, T.K. (1994) 'Race, ethnicity, and class: An analysis of interrelations.' *International Social Science Journal 46*, 1, 83–93.

Parrack, S. and Joseph, G.M. (2007) 'The informal caregivers of aboriginal seniors: Perspectives and issues.' *First Peoples Child and Family Review 3*, 4, 106–113.

Pollitt, P.A. (1996) 'Dementia in old age: An anthropological perspective.' *Psychological Medicine 26*, 5, 1061–1074.

Pollitt, P.A. (1997) 'The problem of dementia in Australian Aboriginal and Torres Strait Islander communities.' *International Journal of Geriatric Psychiatry 12*, 155–163.

Ramsden, I. (2005) 'Towards Cultural Safety.' In D. Wepa (ed.) *Cultural Safety in Aotearoa New Zealand.* Auckland: Pearson Education New Zealand.

Reading, J., Kmetic, A. and Gideon, V. (2007, April) *First Nations Wholistic Policy and Planning Model.* AFN Discussion paper for the World Health Organization Commission on Social Determinants of Health. Ottawa, ON: Assembly of First Nations.

Reid, D., Ryan, T. and Enderby, P. (2001) 'What does it mean to include people with dementia?' *Disability and Society 16*, 3, 377–392.

Searight, H.R. and Gafford, J. (2005) 'Cultural diversity at the end of life: Issues and guidelines for family physicians.' *American Family Physician 71*, 3, 515–522.

Seymour, J., Gott, M., Bellamy, G., Ahmedzai, S.H. and Clarke, D. (2004) 'Planning for the end of life: The views of older people about advance care statements.' *Social Science and Medicine 59*, 1, 57–68.

Smith, D., Varcoe, C. and Edwards, N. (2005) 'Turning around the intergenerational impact of residential schools on aboriginal people: Implications for health policy and practice.' *Canadian Journal of Nursing Research 37*, 4, 38–60.

Solomon, L.D. (2001) *The Jewish Tradition and Choices at the End of Life: A New Judaic Tradition to Illness and Dying.* Lanham, MA: University Press of America.

Stiegelbauer, S.M. (1996) 'What is an elder? What do elders do? First Nations elders as teachers in culture-based urban organizations.' *Canadian Journal of Native Studies 16*, 1, 37–66.

Waid, L.D. and Frazier, L.D. (2003) 'Cultural differences in possible selves in later life.' *Journal of Aging Studies 17*, 251–268.

Wepa, D. (ed.) (2005) *Cultural Safety in Aotearoa New Zealand.* Auckland: Pearson Education New Zealand.

Wepa, D. (2007, 7 December) Keynote presentation at the Cultural Safety Symposium, Westbank, BC.

Widdershoven, G.A.M. and Berghams, R.L.P. (2001) 'Advance directives in dementia care: From instructions to instruments.' *Patient Education and Counseling 44*, 179–186.

PART 2

Policy and
Practice Issues

CHAPTER 7

Decisions, Decisions…

Linking Personalization
to Person-Centred Care

JILL MANTHORPE

Multitudes in the valley of decision.
(*Book of Joel, Old Testament, iii, 14*)

This chapter presents an overview of current issues and developments related to understanding decision-making among people who have dementia in England and Wales. It does this in the context of moves in England to greater personalization of social care and other public services. The chapter gives an outline of the scope of the Mental Capacity Act 2005 (MCA), considers some of the implications of the MCA for community-based practitioners around the areas of planning and working with others in new roles, and interrogates at each step some of the interfaces with moves to the personalization of social care. Practice issues and case vignettes arising out of the MCA in light of the current focus on personalized support are illustrated in five areas: planning ahead; recording; providing information; working with others in new roles; and safeguarding people with dementia. The chapter concludes that the potential for person-centred practice in dementia care will need to be supported by practitioner reflection and service monitoring as much as by the courts and clinicians (Liddle and Johnson 2007).

INTRODUCTION

Support for decision-making

As far back as the Middle Ages in England, in attempts to protect the property and money of people lacking the ability to manage them, the law distinguished between 'natural fools' incapacitated from birth and others who should 'happen to fail of his wit' (Hunt and Phillips 1939). Towards the end of the 20th century, these long-established and largely unchanged proxy decision-making systems regarding finance, health and welfare in England and Wales were proving problematic. Practitioners, families and campaigning groups complained of their complexities and inadequacies, and they did so in greater force because the numbers of people with dementia, in particular, were rising (Age Concern 1986; Law Commission 1995). The problems and uncertainties in dealing with decision-making were most frequently addressed by use of common law (Williamson 2007) and, in practice, systems used varied considerably (Means and Langan 1996). The extent of problems and growing worries about exploitation and financial abuse, in particular, necessitated a solution. This would have to be one that would be acceptable to judicial and administrative systems, to practitioners, to carers – whose views were strongly represented, for example, by the Alzheimer's Society – and to the wider public as taxpayers and citizens. The Enduring Powers of Attorney Act 1985 went some way towards addressing concerns by allowing a person to appoint an attorney to manage his or her financial affairs in the event of future incapacity. However, this did not cover medical or personal care decisions. This meant that people could not appoint a trusted individual to ensure that their wishes in more general areas (e.g. where they might live or consent to a clinical procedure) were carried out when they were no longer in a position to make these known or to give or withhold consent.

The recommendations of the Law Commission (1995) and Making Decisions Alliance (a coalition of voluntary, statutory and professional organizations) to review the law governing the care and treatment of people who lack capacity eventually culminated in the Mental Capacity Act 2005, which came into force in 2007. The Act and accompanying Code of Practice (Department for Constitutional Affairs 2007) reflect and clarify common or existing case law (Dunn *et al.* 2007). New safeguards and practitioner roles, revised organizational structures and fresh paperwork (forms) have been established. Much of this has been done through consultation with professional groups and communities of interest including care providers, advocacy groups and organizations representing people with dementia and their carers. Thus while the legislation and the Code of Practice are definitive, accessible summaries were required for professional and public readerships, together with training materials designed for frontline practitioners (Manthorpe, Rapaport and Stanley 2008). These illustrate the multi-layers of implementation of policy and legislation, the investment required and the diverse audiences that need to be addressed when supporting people with dementia in making decisions. The range includes people seeking to plan for their possible futures; professionals fearing legal challenge (Jackson and Warner 2002); practitioners working in emergency situations, such as ambulance crew (Evans, Warner and Jackson 2008); unqualified practitioners working in unfamiliar territories where what is in a person's best interests may not be obvious (Nazarko 2007); and informal supporters or carers making decisions in climates of conflict or uncertainty.

England and Wales are not alone in addressing these problems through specific legislation. In South Australia there is the Guardianship and Administration Act 1993; the Substitute Decision Act 1992 and the Health Care Consent Act 1996 operate in Ontario, Canada; and, in Scotland, the Adults with Incapacity Act 2000 covers similar groups (Dunn *et al.* 2007). While these Acts are not confined to people with suspected or recognized dementia, this has been a major spur. Wilkinson (2001), for example, observed that the growing emphasis on early diagnosis of dementia led to strong pressure on the Scottish legal system, prompting reform.

Personalization

Parallel to the debate over decision-making has been a growing emphasis on choice and control for citizens in areas that have traditionally been professionally led. In England and Wales over the last two decades, social care (often referred to earlier as community care) has been based on the idea that support should be individualized or closely tailored, responsive and flexible, and reflected in the term 'package of care' coming from a combination of family, friends and public sector and private providers. By the 1990s, care managers developed individual care plans, based on assessments which ideally took full account of each service user's wishes, needs and circumstances.

The limitations of this approach have been recognized as stemming not so much from these ideas and ideals but arising from the rationing of care that is targeted at those in most need; from the general tension of stretching finite resources to meet rising demand; and from problems with the supply of good-quality care. To meet some of these criticisms, made loudly by younger people with disabilities, Direct Payments (DPs) were introduced in 1997. Here, people eligible for social care services, after assessment, are given the money to pay for their own social care, along lines proposed by them and discussed with their care manager. This enables user choice to flourish. Direct Payments have not been available for some people with dementia, because they have not been able to consent to this system (although carers can sometimes receive DPs on their own behalf), but legislation is set to change in this area.

Experimentally, the Individual Budgets (IB) system – which may involve bringing together assessments made by a number of agencies (e.g. those providing social care and those providing equipment) – results in the transparent or explicit allocation of resources to an individual, in cash or in kind, to be spent in ways which suit them. Again, legal safeguards about people who are not able to make decisions over such areas mean that these are limited at the time of writing for people with dementia but the direction of travel in social care is clear (Department of Health 2007). Care will be increasingly personalized and 'personal budgets' for each individual using publicly funded social care services will render more explicit the budget available, the way it has been calculated, and the goals or outcomes that it is intended to meet. Two elements have not gone away in this new system. These include the high threshold for eligibility for services (Commission for Social Care Inspection 2008) and the continuance of means testing for social care support, which differentiates it from health care that is free. The former means that many people with dementia may not be eligible for services because their needs are met by family or are not 'high' enough to meet criteria. The second point gives rise to assumptions that public services are not available for people who have income or savings over and above minimum levels (Henwood and Hudson 2008). However, personal budgets for people with dementia will facilitate wider choices. As we shall see, this places decision-making about care centre stage.

Systems of self-directed support are not confined to the UK (Social Care Institute for Excellence 2007). Similar developments in care systems in other countries are called 'consumer-directed care', 'self-directed support', 'personalized allocations', 'cash for care', and so on (see Glendinning and Kemp 2006 for examples from Europe; Mahoney *et al.* 2004 for examples from the United States). In England people are likely to be able to choose from a continuum of options, with key decisions controlled by the service user, their proxy decision-maker, or by a professional on their behalf. Underpinning these moves are twofold familiar pressures: consumer demand for greater autonomy; and efforts to reduce or contain public expenditure by transferring to consumers or their circles of support, such as families, elements of public service provision (e.g. dealing with the day-to-day business of domiciliary care, from recruitment of staff to dealing with time sheets and payments, to supplementing staff if they do not turn up or leave work unfinished). Squaring this circle is not an easy task.

Respect for people's choices, autonomy and well-being, often summed up as person-centredness, is frequently voiced as a priority by dementia care practitioners, and the new personalization agenda fits well with these values. People with dementia are being equipped with more information and more choices, and in the English context, as elsewhere in the developed world, services are being redesigned so that people are more able to plan or design their own support with public funds (Department of Health 2007). Some commentators have argued that what we are witnessing is part of processes of privatizing or individualizing risk (Ferguson 2007) in the guise of personalizing care. Others see it as a real chance to put person-centred care into practice.

MENTAL CAPACITY ACT 2005 AND PERSONALIZATION

The MCA enshrined much of the practice espoused by people who seek to undertake person-centred care for people with dementia. It set out a framework about what is lawful when making decisions on behalf of people who lack the ability to make specific decisions. It was designed to enhance personal autonomy, and it clarified the extent and legalities of options open to people who wish to make advance decisions about care and treatment or to appoint decision-makers on their behalf. It introduced new proxy decision-making roles to address health, welfare and financial matters, and also enabled specialist advocacy for isolated people for whom major health and welfare decisions are to be made. While the Act is not confined to people with dementia, it is this group of people and their predicaments that were most often envisaged to potentially benefit from the Act. As the description of personalization above suggests, these two areas – empowerment and protection – are likely to engage with each other, for personalization is essentially about choice and control, but if or when a person is no longer able to make decisions then the MCA provides a framework for someone else to make decisions on his or her behalf based on that person's best interests.

The Act is underpinned by five core principles set out in section 1 of the Act and in the Code of Practice (Department for Constitutional Affairs 2007). These are summarized below:

- An assumption of capacity: a lack of capacity to make a decision has to be clearly determined.

- The right to be supported to make a decision: a person must be given appropriate help before a conclusion is reached that he or she cannot make the decision.

- The right to make an unwise or eccentric decision: an unwise decision does not necessarily mean that a person lacks capacity to make it.

- If it is determined that a person lacks capacity to make a decision, any decision on his or her behalf must be in his or her best interests.

- Anything done for or on behalf of people without capacity should be in a way that is less restrictive of their basic rights and freedoms.

These principles must be considered in any assessment of an individual's capacity to make a decision. The Act sets out a clear 'decision-specific' test for assessing whether a person lacks capacity to make a particular decision. It provides a checklist of factors (Part 1, section 4) that must be taken into account in deciding what is in the person's best interests. This means that written or oral statements made by a person must be considered and carers and family members should be consulted by professionals. There are no specified professional groups designated for the role of assessors of capacity, and so any practitioner may be involved in assessing whether a person has capacity to make a specific decision on the basis of the concerns they have identified or others have brought to their attentions (Code of Practice 4.35). The person who assesses the capacity of an individual should be the person directly concerned with the decision (e.g. a surgeon will decide if a patient has the capacity to consent to an operation). As most decisions often involve care, it is family or care workers who are frequently in this position. Professionals or the Court of Protection (the body that may be called upon if no arrangements are made or there are conflicts or uncertainties) may become involved when there are issues arising that care workers or families find problematic or where they are uncertain what to do. Such a framework is helpful for people who work in a person's own home and outside a large organization where there are managers on hand or professionals easily available. Personalization may mean that people with dementia wish to take part more in ordinary activities, such as going shopping, and less often to facilities such as day care centres. We will not know what people prefer until they have greater options for choice. This applies to family carers too, as they may want to take up new forms of short breaks, instead of the traditional offers of day care or 'sitters'. For example, one carer, Katherine, uses the money from Direct Payments to pay a support worker to take her mother to the park to feed the ducks and watch children playing: 'This is a break for me but I can only feel good about it if I know that my mother is not distressed at being separated.'

This new Court of Protection, which can be the final arbiter in the event of disputes, presides over the whole Act. The Office of the Public Guardian registers Lasting Powers of Attorney (see below) and appoints deputies. It is charged, with other agencies, to respond to concerns raised about people undertaking these roles. The Act brought into force new criminal offences to protect people who lack capacity to make decisions from ill treatment or wilful neglect, a subject of increasing interest in both the UK recently (O'Keeffe *et al.* 2007) and Canada (see O'Connor and Donnelly, this volume). This measure may be reassuring for those people with doubts about the higher risks of personalization, where greater choice may leave people more vulnerable to exploitation.

Acting in a person's best interests must underpin decision-making on another's behalf. The requirement to facilitate individual decision-making (MCA section 1) has direct relevance for people with dementia when considering decisions about day-to-day matters such as welfare, care or treatment. Most practice decisions concern ordinary day-to-day decisions in respect to care and treatment although it is often examples about life and death decisions that make the headlines. As this chapter notes, the two parallel agendas of empowerment, but also of protection, may converge.

Planning ahead

Under the MCA a person may appoint one or several attorneys to make decisions in respect of specified welfare, healthcare and financial decisions when they are no longer able to make these independently. The advantages of making these arrangements for a Lasting Power of Attorney (LPA) are that they offer an opportunity for choice and reassurance or peace of mind. The person making an LPA chooses who the attorney will be and the extent of their powers. For professionals working with people with early or suspected dementia, this means that their role in providing information is crucial to avoid missing the opportunity to make decisions around future planning. Information needs to be communicated to individuals and also to family members. Often in the past people with dementia have not received adequate information, and carers frequently report that information for them has never been supplied or coordinated (Glasby and Kilbride 2003). For example, Andrew, another carer, found that he had missed out on tax relief that is reclaimable when buying incontinence pads for a disabled person: 'Only when the pharmacist asked me why I was paying full price did I discover that we could get this taken off the price.'

The LPA may help ensure that care is personalized should a person develop dementia and be unable to make decisions on their own behalf. Some of the decisions facing a person holding an LPA may be significant, such as selling the family home, buying costly equipment, or making alterations to the home. Other decisions may be less substantial in scale but just as supportive, such as signing the contract for a telephone alarm system or paying a home care agency or a neighbour to do the garden. It is not that these activities are new, but for many people they can be complex and previous proxy decision-making only applied to money. For people with dementia and others, decisions about welfare, such as where a person lives, or health care, such as giving consent to treatment, have often seemed to take them on uncertain journeys. Carers, in particular, have frequently commented that professionals seem to hide behind 'confidentiality' principles and that it has been very difficult to find out what is going on. As a third example, June, a family carer, reported recently:

> I rang social services to find out what care they were providing to my parents-in-law as we just could not find out from them [parents-in-law]. We go round regularly but we did not know who was coming in or when. The social worker said she would need to phone my parents-in-law but that was no good, they could not understand what she was talking about, and they don't answer the phone as they are too deaf!

Recording

Records in respect of older people using social and healthcare services vary in terms of what they say and how much use they are. Preston-Shoot and Wigley (2002) identified many gaps in social work records about older service users, finding that they often missed key information. The importance of all practitioners keeping records about any statements of preferences and of the existence of advance decisions and proxy decision-makers chosen by a person is even more important now that the MCA is in place, not least because attorneys and others have rights to see professional records. Information will also be helpful in the event of any disagreements. More widely, those supporting people with dementia at early stages can help them to say what they will want for the future, what is important to them, and to express any beliefs, preferences or values. Who will know, for example, that a person loved animals if their friends and family are no longer around? Who will remember that one person was happy listening to jazz while another preferred brass bands? Who will be able to recall that a person has a religious conviction or its opposite? Other wishes may lie in the area of health care. Decisions about refusing treatment are important to document and to know about. Effective personalized care does not mean that just because a person and their family may have greater control over arranging care, these matters can be ignored. Speaking to this issue, Barbara, an older adult spoken to in preparation of this chapter, notes that she has alerted her younger family members to her advance decisions as well as her siblings: 'None of them are getting younger, and goodness knows which of us will be *compos mentis* when decisions have to be made.'

Information

The MCA requires greater attention to information, communication and recording. Will this lead to an increase in bureaucracy? UK geriatricians' experiences of patients who made living wills prior to the MCA were that these made decision-making clearer for the care team, and that discussion with patients and relatives about end-of-life care was easier if such documents existed (Schiff *et al.* 2006). Whether people will want to think about advance decisions at times when they are discussing diagnosis is debatable – it is thought that many people might find this too early and too soon. Beyond this, there are many implications of advance decisions, notably the potential for people to decide to refuse hospital or invasive treatment, consequently remaining at home or in care homes. There is evidence from the United States that people who draw up documents such as living wills are likely to die at home if this is what they specified (Degenholtz, Rhee and Arnold 2004), and from the UK that nursing home residents are less likely to be moved to hospital if they have a living will indicating that this is *not* what they wanted (Molloy *et al.* 2000).

Mason and Wilkinson (2002) looked at the characteristics of a sample of 62 people with dementia in Scotland and found that 46 (74%) had made a will prior to diagnosis of dementia and seven (11%) made one after receiving the diagnosis; 33 (53%) had given Power of Attorney to someone; and nine (15%) had made arrangements for someone else to deal with their pensions and similar income. However, they also found that the time of diagnosis was often a lost opportunity for passing on information about such matters and that there was a lack of follow-up about whether people had taken in any information that was provided at the time. Moreover, carers were often left with all the burdens of responsibility without corresponding levels of authority, a worrying situation that was frequently unnecessary. The challenge for services, these researchers suggested, is to produce accessible information, but if they are to do this and to communicate information confidently, then professionals need to have knowledge and awareness themselves. In their view, local areas need specialists to coordinate information and support for people with dementia; others might argue that this should be the role of professionals in dementia services overall.

Greater personalization will also require some change to recording and information systems. While the ethos of the approach is to free up creativity and to empower individuals and families, public money responsibilities include accountability and probity. The risks of personalization are being explored through adult protection systems. In England, these are extensive and include national databases for checking to see if potential staff or volunteers have criminal records. These have to be supplemented by knowledge of local risk factors, such as groups or individuals who are targeting vulnerable people, and robust referral processes to enable safeguards to be put in place if there appears to be neglect, exploitation or mistreatment. Concerns over such risks are often high and are international. Evidence from the United States (Simon-Rusinowitz *et al.* 2000, 2002) is that policy experts were concerned about abuse and exploitation but were also mindful of the risk that over-regulation could undermine the empowerment principles of consumer-directed support. Provincial legislation in British Columbia, Canada (Adult Guardianship Act 2000), has attempted to address these concerns, and in England the dilemma of risk versus safeguarding is similarly expressed (Manthorpe, Stevens *et al.* 2008). Karen, for example, another carer who was contacted in preparation for this chapter, indicates that she is worried that her cousin trusts people far too easily and may no longer have so many professionals looking out for her from the day centre, the meals service or the homecare agency, now that she is reliant on one homecare worker.

Working with people in new roles

Both the MCA and personalization mean that people with dementia and carers, as well as practitioners, are taking on new roles. These have the potential to ease conflict, or to reduce uncertainty, but they also may render relationships less clear. They may require some renegotiation about the roles of professionals and patient/client/service user or a person with dementia. White and Baldwin (2006) predict that 'most of the problems that arise out of the Act will be as a result of disagreement between doctors and newly empowered third parties (donees, deputies and IMCAs [see below]) concerning the continuation or discontinuation of specific medical therapies' (p.388). While this may be so in relation to medical treatments, in other areas of life disagreement may well arise between professionals, between professionals and people with dementia and their supporters, and lastly between people with dementia and their families.

In focusing on just one of these new roles, the MCA set up provision for Independent Mental Capacity Advocates (IMCAs) to be instructed to support a person who has no one outside the care team to speak on his or her behalf, in situations where serious medical treatment or change of accommodation decisions are to be made and the person lacks the capacity to make these. Local authorities have further discretionary powers to instruct an IMCA to represent the interests of individuals who have no one else to speak for them other than paid staff in respect of care reviews, and where they are supported (funded) by the local authority or NHS body, and also for adult protection cases, irrespective of whether families, friends and others are involved. (In Wales, the role of IMCAs also extends to cover accommodation reviews and adult protection cases.) Practitioners have to establish ways of working with IMCAs and to accept the shifts in advocacy and negotiation roles. While IMCAs are not decision-makers, their roles are to 'challenge decision-makers assertively' and to coordinate a range of possible viewpoints from multi-professional staff. They are entitled to access records and interview the person in private. Other practitioners will need to avoid duplication of tasks with IMCAs and professional defensiveness. Working with non-instructed advocates (in that the service user will not necessarily have requested the input of an advocate, understand its meaning or be able to communicate) sets up new relationships between professionals and advocates; mutual understandings will need to be fostered. Everyone, it seems, wants to be person-centred.

The role of IMCAs has been welcomed as the first statutory right to advocacy (Rapaport *et al.* 2006), but it is limited. It will not negate the need for practitioners to advocate on behalf of people with dementia, who are frequently marginalized. We have little knowledge of how other people in the galaxy of new workers will combine to support people with dementia. *Service brokers*, for example, working for user-controlled organizations or as independent businesses, may specialize in certain health conditions or they may offer to organize care packages for people from certain ethno-cultural groups, gay and lesbian disabled people, or those living in a rural area. If, as generally predicated, people use personal budgets to employ *personal assistants*, then what training will they receive and from whom? Will professionals have new roles in offering training? How will they relate to *paid family members*, whose work sometimes may not really be very good and not person-centred?

Safeguarding people with dementia under the MCA

On the opposite side of the same coin to the principles of empowerment are rights to be protected or safeguarded. The risks of abuse and neglect for people with dementia are frequently observed, and personalization may heighten these risks. The MCA, on the other hand, offers new elements that may safeguard their well-being. Much will depend on the quality of evidence, the ways in which practitioners and others share information, and how they listen to people with dementia and observe what is going on. Practitioners' records are likely to play a key role here, both in detailing injuries, behaviours or harm, but also in providing evidence in defence of people who have been accused in situations where there has been no abuse. Those working with people with dementia are aware of both their vulnerability to abuse but also the frequent vulnerability of people who are caring for them, often alone and struggling to manage behaviour that is challenging.

Much of this area covers the theme of *risk*, and if we accept that opportunities to plan care and treatment are a breakthrough in empowering people to make important personal decisions, then extra risk is inevitable. While professionals might not agree with people's choices, they have rights to be wrong. However, like other commentators in social care (e.g. Scourfield 2005), many professionals are alert to the difficulty that calculating risks presents to people with dementia. They may face accusations that they are not being person-centred if they raise such matters, and will have to think deeply about what it means to be acting in a person's best interests and why.

CONCLUSION

The principles underpinning the MCA have the potential to influence good practice in the delivery of social care and health services to people with dementia and their carers. Whilst the MCA has been largely welcomed (see Alzheimer's Society 2007), there are needs to raise public awareness, provide training for staff, and build up effective monitoring arrangements, as well as to provide opportunities to debate the working of it in practice and workforce capacity. Likewise, personalization is welcomed, though, as we have seen, professionals are troubled by the potential for people who are not able to defend themselves to be exploited or mistreated.

The procedures of the MCA and greater ability to make choices about future care and treatment have the potential to enhance effective practice, and thus contribute to person-centred autonomy and empowerment. There are likely to be key transitions when advice and assistance may be most beneficial, such as at the time of diagnosis or planning care. Professionals may need to devote time to assist people with dementia and their carers to benefit from the Act, and to make sure that they have accessible explanations for people to read and discuss. In the future, people with dementia and carers may be better informed and more confident. Good practice should not remain in pockets. We know little about how to create or facilitate learning- and change-oriented cultures within health and social care organizations, and the systemic capacity to introduce new ways of thinking, learning and working appears to be lacking (McDonnell and Ferlie 2002).

There are no 'magic bullets' for improving the quality of dementia care, and methods for changing professional behaviour are poorly developed and understood. Processes of change are complex and slow, require different skills at different stages, and are dependent on contextual factors, particularly in the local environment (Hughes *et al.* 2002). This means that we should be looking for changes from the MCA to evolve from making better decisions to transforming how decisions are made and for personalization's impacts to be steady rather than instantly transformational. In England, the two changes are being implemented at much the same time, and this chapter has explored ways in which they interrelate throughout the journey of a person with dementia.

REFERENCES

Age Concern (1986) *The Law and Vulnerable Elderly People.* London: Age Concern.

Alzheimer's Society (2007) 'The right to decide.' *The National Newsletter of the Alzheimer's Society*, March, 12–13.

Commission for Social Care Inspection (2008) *The State of Social Care in England 2006–07.* London: Commission for Social Care Inspection.

Degenholtz, H., Rhee, Y. and Arnold, R. (2004) 'Brief communication: The relationship between having a living will and dying in place.' *Annals of Internal Medicine 141*, 113–117.

Department for Constitutional Affairs (2007) *Mental Capacity Act 2005 Code of Practice.* Norwich: The Stationery Office. Available online at www.justice.gov.uk/guidance/mca-code-of-practice.htm, accessed 14 November 2008.

Department of Health (2007) *Putting People First.* London: The Stationery Office.

Dunn, M. Clare, I., Holland, A.J. and Gunn, M. (2007) 'Constructing and reconstructing "best interests": An interpretive examination of substitute decision-making under the Mental Capacity Act 2005.' *Journal of Social Welfare and Family Law 29*, 2, 117–133.

Evans, K., Warner, J. and Jackson, E. (2008) 'How much do emergency healthcare workers know about capacity and consent?' *Emergency Medicine Journal 24*, 391–393.

Ferguson, I. (2007) 'Increasing user control or privatizing risk? The antinomies of personalization.' *British Journal of Social Work 37*, 387–403.

Glasby, J. and Kilbride, L. (2003) 'Who knows? The provision of information to the carers of people with dementia.' *Practice 15*, 4, 51–67.

Glendinning, C. and Kemp, P. (eds) (2006) *Cash and Care: Policy Challenges in the Welfare State.* Bristol: The Policy Press.

Henwood, M. and Hudson, B. (2008) *Lost to the System? The Impact of Fair Access to Care.* London: Commission for Social Care Inspection.

Hughes, J., Humphrey, C., Rogers, S. and Greenhalgh, T. (2002) *Evidence into Action: Changing Practice in Primary Care*. London: Royal College of General Practitioners.

Hunt, D. and Phillips, J. (1939) *Heywood and Massey's Lunacy Practice* (6th edn). London: Stevens and Sons.

Jackson, E. and Warner, J. (2002) 'How much do doctors know about consent and capacity?' *Journal of the Royal Society of Medicine 95*, 601–603.

Law Commission (1995) *Mental Incapacity*. London: HMSO.

Liddle, C. and Johnson, J. (2007) 'The Mental Capacity Act 2005: A new framework for health decision making.' *Journal of Medical Ethics 33*, 94–97.

Mahoney, K.J., Simon-Rusinowitz, L., Loughlin, D.M., Desmond, S.M. and Squillace, M. (2004) 'Determining personal care consumers' preferences for a consumer-directed cash and counselling option: Survey results from Arkansas, Florida, New Jersey and New York elders and adults with physical disabilities.' *Health Service Research 39*, 3, 643–664.

Manthorpe, J., Rapaport, J. and Stanley, N. (2008) 'The Mental Capacity Act 2005 and its influences on social work practice: Debate and synthesis.' *Practice 20*, 3, 151–162.

Manthorpe, J., Stevens, M., Rapaport, J., Harris, J. *et al.* (2008) 'Safeguarding and system change: Early perceptions of the implications for adult protection services of the English Individual Budget pilots – A qualitative study.' *British Journal of Social Work*. Advance Access published online 26 March 2008.

Mason, A. and Wilkinson, H. (2002) *The Characteristics of People with Dementia Who Are Users and Non-Users of the Legal System: A Feasibility Study*. Edinburgh: Scottish Executive Social Research. Available online at www.scotland.gov.uk/Resource/Doc/46932/0013927.pdf, accessed 14 November 2008.

McDonnell, J. and Ferlie, E. (2002) 'Towards high change, high learning organisations in primary care.' *Department of Health Primary Care Research Bulletin 2*, 16–19.

Means, R. and Langan, J. (1996) 'Money "handling", financial abuse and elderly people with dementia: Implications for welfare professionals.' *Health and Social Care in the Community 4*, 6, 353–358.

Molloy, D., Guyatt, G., Russo, R. and Goeree, R. *et al.* (2000) 'Systematic implementation of an advance directive program in nursing homes: A randomized control trial.' *Journal of the American Medical Association 283*, 1437–1444.

Nazarko, L. (2007) 'The Mental Capacity Act and care documentation.' *Nursing and Residential Care 9*, 5, 227–229.

O'Keeffe, M., Hills, A., Doyle, M., McCreadie, C. *et al.* (2007) *UK Study of Abuse and Neglect of Older People: Prevalence Survey Report*. London: National Centre for Social Care Research.

Preston-Shoot, M. and Wigley, V. (2002) 'Closing the circle: social workers' responses to multi-agency procedures on older age abuse.' *British Journal of Social Work 32*, 3, 299–320.

Rapaport, J., Manthorpe, J., Hussein, S., Moriarty, J. and Collins, J. (2006) 'Old issues and new directions: Perceptions of advocacy, its extent and effectiveness from a qualitative study of stakeholder views.' *Journal of Intellectual Disabilities 10*, 2 191–210.

Schiff, R., Sacares, P., Snook, J., Chakravarthi, R. and Bulpitt, C. (2006) 'Living wills and the Mental Capacity Act: A postal questionnaire survey of UK geriatricians.' *Age and Ageing 35*, 116–121.

Scourfield, P. (2005) 'Implementing the Community Care (Direct Payments) Act: Will the supply of personal assistants meet the demand and at what price?' *Journal of Social Policy* *34*, 469–488.

Simon-Rusinowitz, L., Bochniak, A.M., Mahoney, K.J., Marks, L.N. and Hecht, D. (2000) 'Implementation issues for consumer directed programs: A survey of policy experts.' *Generations 24*, 1, 34–40.

Simon-Rusinowitz, L., Marks, L.N., Loughlin, D.M., Desmond, S.M. *et al.* (2002) 'Implementation issues for consumer-directed programs: Competing views of policy experts, consumers and representatives.' *Journal of Aging and Social Policy 14*, 3/4, 95–118.

Social Care Institute for Excellence (2007) *Choice, Control and Individual Budgets: Emerging Themes*. London: Social Care Institute for Excellence.

White, M. and Baldwin, T. (2006) 'The Mental Capacity Act 2005 – Implications for anaesthesia and critical care.' *Anaesthesia 61*, 381–389.

Wilkinson, H. (2001) 'Empowerment and decision-making for people with dementia: The use of legal interventions in Scotland.' *Aging and Mental Health 5*, 4, 322–328.

Williamson, T. (2007) 'Capacity to protect – The Mental Capacity Act explained.' *Journal of Adult Protection 9*, 1, 25–32.

CHAPTER 8

Confronting the Challenges of Assessing Capacity
Dementia in the Context of Abuse[1]

DEBORAH O'CONNOR AND MARTHA DONNELLY

Mary Wilson is an 82-year-old woman suffering from emphysema and severe arthritis. She also demonstrates signs of early dementia including poor short-term memory, disorientation to time and location, and impaired insight. Prior to her recent hospitalization, she lived with her husband of over 50 years and was dependent upon him for assistance with all of her daily care needs. His ability to provide this care is questionable – he is unable to establish reasonable routines for her care, prevents her from having contact with others, is routinely overheard by neighbours verbally berating her, and is physically rough with her. Several months ago, Mrs Wilson was admitted to the hospital in very poor physical condition – she was confused, emaciated and dehydrated. She improved dramatically and, against the advice of the healthcare team, she returned to her apartment under the care of her husband. Both refused all home supports but did co-operate with periodic visits from the family physician. Recently, during one of these visits, Mrs Wilson was found once again to be dehydrated, malnourished and very weak; she requested that she be taken to the hospital. Her condition is now stabilized and her husband is insistent that she return home. Mrs Wilson indicates that she is quite frightened by her husband and does not believe he can take care of her. However, she is not agreeing to remain in care nor will she agree to a restraining order against Mr Wilson even though he is becoming belligerent and threatening.

People with dementia are more vulnerable to situations of abuse and neglect. On the one hand, increasing dependency on others and deteriorating social networks leave the person more isolated, creating a context that is ripe for becoming abusive. Simultaneously, cognitive difficulties interfere with the ability to take action – for example, the person may have difficulty organizing to leave or seek support.

Health professionals attempting to deal with these situations are commonly forced to assess the decision-making capacity of the person with dementia as they attempt to establish a balance between rights to autonomy and needs for protection. Despite the apparent and pragmatic link between abuse and capacity, however, surprisingly little attention has been given to examining decision-making capacity within a context of abuse. For example, a recent literature search of major databases including PsycLit, Sociofile, ERIC and OVID using keywords which combined abuse and/or neglect with capacity and/or competence assessments revealed only one actual hit (Dong and Gorbein 2005). Similarly, keyword searches of several popular texts on assessing competence did not address how situations of abuse might influence the assessments (see for example Grisso and Applebaum 1998; White 1994). Articles related to abuse do note the need to assess capacity when services are being refused (see for example Lachs and Pillemer 2004), but they routinely fail to move beyond this directive to make explicit what this assessment would look like. This is a particularly pertinent gap in the field of dementia studies.

The purpose of this chapter is to begin to highlight the need to consider the importance of context – particularly in situations of abuse – in both undertaking assessments and making determinations about capacity. The plan is to bring together two relatively disparate bodies of literature – the abuse literature and the literature around assessing decision-making capacity – in order to examine how they may intersect. It is hoped that by drawing attention to this one context, the complexity associated with the assessment process in general will be demonstrated. It is suggested that, by attending to this context, personhood issues can be addressed in the assessment process.

EXAMINING THE ELDER ABUSE LITERATURE

Internationally, elder abuse is increasingly recognized as an important health and social problem (Krug *et al.* 2002). Elder abuse generally, but not always, encapsulates three main concepts: (1) intentional actions that (2) cause harm or create serious risk of harm to (3) vulnerable elders (Lachs and Pillemer 2004). In Canada, general prevalence studies suggest that approximately 4 per cent of seniors experience abuse or neglect (Podnieks 1992) while international figures range between 2 and 10 per cent (Thomas 2000). At least some of this variance is undoubtedly related to different ways of defining abuse and the research methods used. Some groups have been identified as being at greater risk – for example, one study found that about 20 per cent of clients on a psycho-geriatric service met the criteria for abuse (Vida, Monks and Des Rosiers 2002) and several other studies have identified a much higher prevalence of physical abuse when one spouse has dementia (Buttell 1999; O'Connor 1999). Financial abuse is generally identified as the most common form of abuse perpetrated against seniors, although there is some suspicion that, at least in part, this finding may be because it is easier to recognize and less heavily shrouded in silence compared to other forms of family violence.

Within the literature there has been a relatively strong focus on developing victim and abuser profiles. It is becoming increasingly clear, though, that there is not one particular picture of 'an abuser' – rather this person looks different depending upon the type of abuse. For example, spouses (husbands in particular) are most likely to abuse physically, while strangers or offspring are more likely to perpetrate financial or resource abuse. There is, however, some consensus that the abuser is more likely to be male (as summarized by Penhale 2003) and/or have mental health issues and/or experience drug/alcohol problems and dependency issues (Lachs and Pillemer 2004). Attempts to uncover a common 'victim' profile have also met with limited success but do reveal some trends. Specifically, although some studies suggest otherwise, most research indicates that women are more likely to be abused (Hightower *et al.* 1999; Penhale 2003). Physical frailty, cognitive impairment and social isolation are identified as risk factors (Barnett, Miller-Perrin and Perrin 2005; Lachs and Pillemer 2004).

Research in this area has been criticized as largely atheoretical (Biggs 2003). When theoretical explanations have been offered, they often draw upon theories such as caregiver stress or intergenerational theory. These perspectives, however, have only limited empirical support and have been critiqued as inadequate (see for example Lachs and Pillemer 2004; Penhale 2003).

Critical feminist theory has more recently been introduced into the elder abuse literature as a potentially more inclusive and powerful lens for conceptualizing the dynamics of abuse. This lens draws attention to two aspects that underpin an understanding of abuse: gender and power (Yllo 2005). It recognizes that abuse is generally about power inequities both within the relationship and society at large. Violence is conceptualized as coercive control, and it is reinforced by societal subordination of some groups over others (Harbison 1999; Whitaker 1995). Most research examining power dynamics in abuse has focused on gender – the reinforcement of male domination and female subordination – but the societal marginalization of aging persons, particularly those who carry the stigma of dementia, is also an important consideration in understanding elder abuse. In other words, although most often applied to women, a critical feminist lens need not just be concerned with females but rather focuses on all persons who are oppressed or marginalized. This lens suggests that, in order to fully conceptualize the dynamics of abuse, emphasis must be given to understanding the nature of power within relationships (Penhale 2003).

A feminist lens draws attention to the importance of social location, including gender, as a critical factor in this experience; it suggests that men and women may differ dramatically in terms of the meanings and interpretations that they accord the abuse, hence it calls for a gender-sensitive analysis of the issues. One way that this can be understood is in relation to psychological development. Specifically, new ways of examining women's psychological and moral development suggest that many women may be more motivated by a focus on relational connection than on a desire for autonomy or self-determination. There is a growing body of research that indicates that women's sense of self is more likely to be developed and defined within her relationships with others – she judges herself and her worth by her ability to develop, maintain and sustain relationships (see for example Gilligan 1982; Jordan et al. 1997; Kaschak 1992). This contrasts with traditional Western understandings of psychological development that suggest that man (sic) is motivated toward increasing autonomy and independence. Thus, a feminist lens highlights the need to take a gender-sensitive lens when trying to understand the subjective experience of the person who is being victimized.

Returning to the case vignette then, the point being made here is that any assessment of Mrs Wilson's capability to participate in a particular decision must take into consideration these two interrelated dynamics of the abusive situation – power and gender. The next step will be to shift the focus to the capacity assessment in order to begin to highlight how each of these might influence what the capacity assessment would look like and how it might be interpreted.

FOREGROUNDING THE ASSESSMENTS OF CAPACITY

Setting the stage for an assessment of capacity requires recognition of four issues. The first is identifying what the assessment of capacity is actually assessing. Since the early 1990s there has been a great deal of discussion about the need to move from general to domain-specific decisions on capability. Although consensus appears to have been reached on the importance of this shift, jurisdictions vary regarding the extent that they have actually adopted this philosophy. In general, at least eight major capacity domains have been established with some requiring a broader set of cognitive and procedural skills than others – for example, independent living and financial capacity are considered broader in scope than testamentary capacity, treatment consent, research consent, sexual consent or voting (Moye and Marson 2007). Much of the research has focused on the less complex domains, especially consent to treatment and research participation, with the focus on independent living receiving the least amount of attention.

While these domains may appear clear, even in similar-sounding situations, what is actually being assessed may vary across jurisdictions. In Canada, for example, both Ontario and British Columbia (BC) have legislation designed to provide guidelines around intervening in situations where a person is living at risk related to abuse or self-neglect. However, what is actually being assessed, and hence what an outcome of incapacity would mean, differs considerably. Specifically, in Ontario, Mrs Wilson might be assessed under the Substitute Decisions Act (SDA) to determine whether or not she was *capable of making decisions about her personal and/or financial care needs*. In contrast, under Part 3 of the Adult Guardianship Act (AGA) in BC, if it were determined that she was being abused or neglected, Mrs Wilson would be assessed to determine whether or not she was *capable of turning down a Support and Assistance Plan (SAP)* being offered by health and social care professionals. Interestingly, if the Mental Health Act were invoked in either province, capacity issues could be entirely bypassed, simply by demonstrating that the person was at risk and had a mental illness (including dementia). This is despite evidence to suggest that presence of a mental illness is not sufficient to predict capacity (Grisso and Appelbaum 1998; Jeste and Saks 2006; Saks and Jeste 2006). Similar inconsistencies are seen both nationally and internationally.

This leads to the second issue, the need to articulate the standards being used to evaluate capacity. Although in their classic article Roth, Meisel and Lidz (1977) initially cited seven standards, more recently these have been narrowed to four: evidencing a choice; understanding relevant information; appreciating the significance of that information for one's own situation; and demonstrating the ability to reason. Different tests of capacity draw on different standards. For example, in BC, the focus would be on Mrs Wilson's *ability to understand* what was being offered, why it was being offered, and possible consequences associated with turning down the SAP. In contrast, she might be assessed quite differently in Ontario where standards more explicitly include both understanding and appreciating. Since appreciation is identified as requiring a higher level of functioning than understanding, presumably it would be more likely that Mrs Wilson would be found not capable in Ontario than in BC. But would she? Although within the legal profession there are fine distinctions between understanding and appreciation, research demonstrates that the boundary between these two is, in practice, not as finite and clear as these definitions would imply (Kim, Karlawish and Caine 2002; Saks and Jeste 2006). Furthermore, it is often health professionals, particularly physicians, who are doing the assessments rather than lawyers, and they may have even less familiarity with the subtle legal distinctions. Finally, the congruence between actual practice and these standards is suspect. While these standards focus on the individual, in practice notions such as 'tolerable risk' – in other words the health professionals' assessment of the situation rather than the person's actual ability to choose – often guide decision-making about capacity. The point here is that standards for assessing capacity differ considerably and need to be articulated, but even when this occurs there remains the possibility that there may still be diverse interpretations.

The third issue, particularly relevant to the focus of this chapter, draws attention to the narrow view that assessments often take. Mental functioning requires at least three functionally distinct, but interactive, systems: intellect, emotionality and control. The intellect is the information-handling system and includes thought processing, perception, orientation, memory, judgment and intelligence; emotionality includes feelings and motivations; and control refers to the expression of behaviour (White 1994). However, although there is some recognition that emotionality and control may interfere with functions of intellect, these aspects have largely been ignored within assessments of capacity. Rather, in most cases, capacity to consent lies exclusively within the domain of intellect, and decisions about it are generally grounded in cognitive tests (Kim *et al.* 2002) while personal and environment-related factors are seen as making potentially important but, as yet, undetermined contributions (Jeste and Saks 2006; see also Moye *et al.* 2007). That this exclusivity and inattention to context and psycho-social factors is problematic becomes quite apparent when abuse is superimposed into this assessment.

Perhaps unsurprisingly, a fourth issue related to understanding capacity is that information about the most appropriate procedures for assessing decision-making capacity is limited (Mullaly *et al.* 2007) and current assessment practices have been critiqued as inadequate (see for example Moye *et al.* 2007). Considerable emphasis has been placed upon developing standardized tests, but apart from identifying general cognitive domains, there is very little information about the specific techniques and processes that should be used for establishing the presence and adequacy of these abilities (Moye *et al.* 2007; Mullaly *et al.* 2007). Often, general purpose tests such as the Mini Mental Status Examination (MMSE) (Folstein, Folstein and McHugh 1975) are used, but while these may link to capacity, there is considerable controversy around their use because they were not developed with the purpose of assessing capacity (see Sullivan 2004 for further discussion of this issue). Other tests more specific to assessing capacity are being developed, but the reliability and validity of these measures has yet to be fully established, particularly in relation to non-medical-related treatment decisions (see for example Dunn *et al.* 2006; Moye and Marson 2007; Moye, Gurrera and Karel 2006; Moye *et al.* 2004; Sullivan 2004).

Combined, these points suggest that the field of knowledge about capacity assessments is still emerging with many challenging questions regarding process and standards yet to be addressed. The implications of these gaps become particularly apparent in more complex situations, such as the assessment of capacity in situations of abuse.

INTEGRATING AN UNDERSTANDING OF ABUSE INTO THE CAPACITY ASSESSMENT

The importance of the psycho-social realm in the assessment and interpretation of capacity emerges as critical in situations of abuse. It offers a context that will differentially influence how the assessment is conducted and findings are interpreted. In order to organize this discussion, the remainder of this chapter will begin to make explicit how issues of power and gender emerging from the abuse literature will influence the assessment process and determination of capacity. This discussion will focus on three aspects – safety, disempowerment and gender-sensitive meaning-making – particularly in relationship to understanding potential consequences.

Safety issues

The most obvious implication associated with conducting assessments of capacity where abuse may be present revolves around the influence of safety considerations on both how the assessment is done and what is said. In relation to conducting the assessment, contradictory directions will be provided depending upon whether one relies upon the abuse literature or capacity literature to direct one's approach. For example, a common piece of advice given to capacity assessors when conducting assessments is to maximize the 'patient's performance' by involving close family or friends to help alleviate anxiety (see for example Grisso and Appelbaum 1998). This advice directly conflicts with best practices associated with interviewing in situations of potential abuse where the common recommendation is that the 'victim' be seen alone in order to ensure that the process affords some protection to him/her.

Implementing an assessment of capacity within a context of potential abuse, then, requires special considerations. These include: Can some level of safety be ensured? Is there space for the person to tell her story in a safe, secure atmosphere? How will the person, competent or not, be protected following the assessment? How can the assessment of capacity integrate a means for considering potential levels of intimidation, prompting and/or 'undue influence'?

Disempowerment

Issues related to powerlessness and futility influence the assessment of capacity in two ways. First, they direct attention to the need to consider the extent that decision-making may be impaired related to a context of disempowerment. Arguably, even when not explicitly stated, a fundamental assumption of most assessments of decision-making capacity is that the person is evidencing a choice. But is s/he able to do this? If not, is this a sign of incapacity or lack of skills and practice? For example, an assessment of incapacity was initiated with Mrs Wilson because, on the surface, she appeared to be turning down the support and assistance plan being offered to her. Further exploration, however, revealed that Mrs Wilson was not actually making a decision to turn down support. Rather, she was refusing to make a decision. This could be tracked to her history of abuse.

> Both the collateral obtained and Mrs Wilson's own stories indicated that she was the victim of a longstanding abusive marital relationship which had destroyed her sense of competence and confidence around independent decision-making. Since her marriage, most control for decision-making had been in the hands of her husband. Moreover, she described incidents of being berated and embarrassed in front of others by her husband, which further eroded her self-confidence. When asked directly she described herself as someone who was not capable of making a decision. As a result, her lack of

support for the health professionals' plan was not based on a decision not to support it, but was rather related to a 'non-decision'.

In order to avoid identifying all abused people as incapable, several more questions appear to be relevant to the assessment of capacity. First, does the person understand that, by not making a decision, s/he is in fact making a decision? Is s/he aware of the potential risks associated with this lack of choice? Alternatively, is the person simply agreeing to something because s/he feels s/he has no power to influence it anyway? And importantly, is s/he able to change her mind at a later date?

> Prior to her hospitalization, Mrs Wilson had essentially been a hostage in her apartment because she was too weak even to reach the phone to call for help. As a result of the care and treatment she was receiving in the hospital, she was now stronger but still dependent upon others for support and assistance. It was unclear if she understood that, without support, she would weaken and once again be vulnerable and unable to mobilize assistance. She had no plans to address this.

In addition to understanding the degree that capacity to make decisions may be influenced by a sense of powerlessness and futility, there is also a need to address power dynamics in the actual assessment. This raises another potential disjuncture between assessment in situations of abuse and neglect, and traditional guidelines around assessing incapacity. Specifically, strategies for ensuring that the assessment process does not further victimize the person being abused, which, though often explicitly addressed in the abuse literature, are missing from the literature focused on assessing capacity. These strategies include taking steps to equalize power dynamics and to establish a trusting relationship between the interviewer and the person who is being abused. The importance of establishing good rapport between the assessor and person being assessed is often described in the literature outlining the assessment process. However, this body of literature provides no explicit direction for addressing the power dynamics between the two parties. Given the 'expert' status typically assigned to the assessor, the assessment process may inadvertently position the person being assessed in a one-down position, effectively disempowering that person and limiting his/her responses.

Gendering understanding of consequences and meaning-making

Two values underpin discussions about assessments of capacity: promotion of well-being and principles of autonomy and self-determination (Grisso and Appelbaum 1998). There is growing recognition that these values may be culturally and gender-biased, based upon Westernized ideals and gender-insensitive developmental models. This means that assessments of capacity may be presupposing motivations and criteria that may be more relevant for some than for others. For example, a relational lens for understanding women's growth and development suggests the need to consider that, for many women, independence/autonomy may not be the driving force around decision-making. Instead, the drive to maintain relational connections may be more pivotal to her well-being.[2]

> Mrs Wilson became quite teary when talking about the dilemma she faced in terms of attending to her own needs versus those of others. She noted that if she agreed to accept the support being suggested, she would be placed in a position where she would be forced to defy her husband. She was ambivalent about doing this. She recognized that the plan might be in her best interest but also voiced fear that this decision would result in her husband carrying out his threat to kill himself if she left. She clearly indicated she would feel responsible if this happened. Moreover, she felt she would be seen by others, including her children, as a 'bad' or selfish person (mother/wife) if she placed her own needs before those of her family – this was totally inconsistent with her perception of herself as a caring person.

In this case, Mrs Wilson was not striving for autonomy and self-determination. These ideals were foreign to her and, consistent with many other women, viewed as 'selfish' (Miller 1987).

This has direct implications for assessing capacity and understanding personal decision-making. It suggests that appreciation of consequences related to a particular decision must move beyond a consideration of threats to individually based independence and autonomy to recognize that, for many women (and undoubtedly others with cultural values that differ from dominant Western society), a sense of well-being is formed in relation to others. Actions that jeopardize this relational connection may be resisted. This means that when exploring 'understanding and appreciation' of potential consequences related to an action (or non-action), an overlooked but critical consequence to consider is how a particular action will influence the abused victim's relational connections and what this means to her sense of self as a 'good' person. For example, given the choice between their own personal safety and protecting their children, many women may choose to refuse assistance. This is related to the shame of acknowledging a relational deficit but also because causing harm to her child may be perceived as more personally devastating to her than being physically hurt.

When principles of autonomy, well-being and self-determination provide the framework for evaluating the rationale of decisions, one set of consequences makes sense. When issues of relational connection are considered, an entirely different set of criteria for understanding consequences emerges. In situations of abuse, the importance of relational connections for helping women define themselves surfaces repeatedly as providing a vital context for understanding their actions, choices and lack of choices. Without this understanding, assessors run the risk of under-evaluating the consequences associated with potentially jeopardizing a relational connection that has been foundational to that person's sense of who she is. This suggests the importance of emotionality in the assessment of capacity, particularly in a context of abuse.

CONCLUSION

Attempting to understand the behaviours and actions of someone within the context of abuse can be challenging. When the person fails to co-operate with health professionals, questions invariably emerge regarding the person's capacity to make decisions. When that person has dementia, it can be even easier to slide into an acceptance of incapacity rather than query difference. One purpose of this chapter has been to demonstrate how and why assessments of capacity must be adapted to take into consideration the dynamics of abuse. The second implicit purpose has been to suggest the importance of broadening the scope of the assessment process as a means for ensuring that assessment moves beyond a focus on intellect to the entire person.

ACKNOWLEDGMENT

This work was supported in part through a Social Sciences and Humanities Research Foundation (SSHRC) Development Research Grant (#820-2006-1030).

ENDNOTES

1. This is an adapted version of the following previously published work: O'Connor, D., Hall, M. and Donnelly, M. (2009) Assessing capacity in the context of Abuse. *Journal of Elder Abuse and Neglect 21 (2)* p.156–169. Used with permission by publisher and all authors.

2. This would be equally applicable to those from cultural backgrounds that place higher value on community and relationships than on independence and autonomy; for instance, those from a traditional South Asian background (see for example Tsai 2001).

REFERENCES

Barnett, O., Miller-Perrin, C. and Perrin, R. (2005) *Family Violence across the Lifespan: An Introduction* (2nd edn). Thousand Oaks, CA: Sage.

Biggs, S. (2003) 'Negotiating Aging Identity: Surface, Depth, and Masquerade.' In J. Hendricks (series ed.) and S. Biggs, A. Lowenstein and J. Hendricks (vol. eds) *The Need for Theory: Critical Approaches to Social Gerontology*. Amityville, NY: Baywood Publishing.

Buttell, F. (1999) 'The relationship between spouse abuse and the maltreatment of dementia sufferers by their caregivers.' *American Journal of Alzheimer's Disease 14*, 4, 230–232.

Dong, X. and Gorbein, M. (2005) 'Decision-making capacity: The core of self-neglect.' *Journal of Elder Abuse and Neglect 17*, 3, 19–36.

Dunn, L., Nowrangi, M., Palmer, B., Jeste, D. and Saks, E. (2006) 'Assessing decisional capacity for clinical research or treatment: A review of instruments.' *American Journal of Psychiatry 163*, 8, 1323–1334.

Folstein, M.F., Folstein, S.E. and McHugh, P.R. (1975) 'Mini-mental status examination: A practical method for grading the cognitive state of patients for the clinician.' *Journal of Psychiatric Research 12*, 189–198.

Gilligan, C. (1982) *In a Different Voice: Psychological Theory and Women's Development*. Cambridge, MA: Harvard University Press.

Grisso, T. and Appelbaum, P.S. (1998) *Assessing Competence to Consent to Treatment: A Guide for Physicians and Other Health Professionals*. New York: Oxford University Press.

Harbison, J. (1999) 'The changing career of "Elder Abuse and Neglect" as a social problem in Canada: Learnings from feminist frameworks?' *Journal of Elder Abuse and Neglect 11*, 4, 59–80.

Hightower, J., Smith, M., Ward-Hall, C. and Hightower, H. (1999) 'Meeting the needs of abused older women? A British Columbia and Yukon transition house survey.' *Journal of Elder Abuse and Neglect 11*, 4, 39–57.

Jeste, D.V. and Saks, E. (2006) 'Decisional capacity in mental illness and substance use disorders: Empirical database and policy implications.' *Behavioral Sciences and the Law 24*, 4, 607–628.

Jordan, J.V., Kaplan, A.G., Miller, J.B., Stiver, I.P. and Surrey, J.L. (1997) *Women's Growth in Connection: Writings from the Stone Center*. New York: Guilford Press.

Kaschak, E. (1992) *Engendered Lives: New Psychology of Women's Experience*. New York: Basic Books.

Kim, Y.H., Karlawish, J.H.T. and Caine, E.D. (2002) 'Current state of research on decision-making competence of cognitively impaired elderly persons.' *American Journal of Geriatric Psychiatry 10*, 2, 151–165.

Krug, E., Dahlberg, L.L., Mercy, J.A., Zwi, A.B. and Lozano, R. (eds) (2002) *World Report on Violence and Health*. Geneva: WHO Press.

Lachs, M.S. and Pillemer, K. (2004) 'Elder abuse.' *The Lancet 364*, 9441, 1263–1272.

Miller, J.B. (1987) *Toward a New Psychology of Women*. New York: Beacon.

Moye, J. and Marson, D.C. (2007) 'Assessment of decision-making capacity in older adults: An emerging area of practice and research.' *Journal of Gerontology Series B: Psychological Sciences and Social Sciences 62B*, 1, P3–P11.

Moye, J., Butz, S.W., Marson, D.C., Wood, E. and the ABA-APA Capacity Assessment of Older Adults Working Group (2007) 'A conceptual model and assessment template for capacity evaluation in adult guardianship.' *Gerontologist 4*, 5, 591–603.

Moye, J., Gurrera, R.J. and Karel, M.J. (2006) 'Empirical advances in the assessment of the capacity to consent to medical treatment: Clinical implications and research needs.' *Clinical Psychology Review 26*, 1054-1077.

Moye, J., Karel, M.J., Azar, A.R. and Gurrera, R.J. (2004) 'Capacity to consent to treatment: Empirical comparison of three instruments in older adults with and without dementia.' *Gerontologist 44*, 2, 166–175.

Mullaly, E., Kinsella, G., Berberovic, N., Cohen, Y. *et al.* (2007) 'Assessment of decision-making capacity: Exploration of common practices among neuropsychologists.' *Australian Psychologist 42*, 3, 78–186.

O'Connor, D.L. (1999) 'Living with a memory-impaired spouse: (Re)Cognizing the experience.' *Canadian Journal on Aging 18*, 2, 211–235.

Penhale, B. (2003) 'Older women, domestic violence and elder abuse: A review of commonalities, differences and shared approaches.' In E. Podnieks, J. Kosberg and A. Lowenstein (eds) *Elder Abuse: Selected Papers from the Prague World Congress on Family Violence*. New York: Haworth Press.

Podnieks, E. (1992) 'National survey of elder abuse in Canada.' *Journal of Elder Abuse and Neglect 4*, 1, 5–58.

Roth, L.H., Meisel, A. and Lidz, C.W. (1977) 'Tests of competency to consent to treatment.' *American Journal of Psychiatry 134*, 279–284.

Saks, E.R. and Jeste, D.V. (2006) 'Capacity to consent to or refuse treatment and/or research: Theoretical considerations.' *Behavioural Sciences and the Law 24*, 411–429.

Sullivan, K. (2004) 'Neuropsychological assessment of mental capacity.' *Neuropsychology Review 14*, 3, 131–142.

Thomas, C. (2000) 'First national study of elder abuse and neglect: Contrast with results from other studies.' *Journal of Elder Abuse and Neglect 12*, 1–14.

Tsai, D.F. (2001) 'How should doctors approach patients? A Confucian reflection on personhood.' *Journal of Medical Ethics 27*, 1, 44–50.

Vida, S., Monks, R.C. and Des Rosiers, P. (2002) 'Prevalence and correlates of elder abuse and neglect in a geriatric psychiatry service.' *Canadian Journal of Psychiatry 47*, 5, 459–467.

Whitaker, T. (1995) 'Violence, gender and elder abuse: Toward a feminist analysis and practice.' *Journal of Gender Studies 4*, 1, 35–45.

White, B.C. (1994) *Competence to Consent*. Washington, DC: Georgetown University Press.

Yllo, K.A. (2005) 'Through a Feminist Lens: Gender Diversity and Violence: Extending the Feminist Framework.' In D. Loseke, R.J. Gelles and M.M. Cavanaugh (eds) *Current Controversies on Family Violence* (2nd edn). Thousand Oaks, CA: Sage.

CHAPTER 9

Capacity, Vulnerability, Risk and Consent

Personhood in the Law

MARGARET ISABEL HALL

INTRODUCTION

Policy makers are increasingly concerned with the protection needs of the *capable but vulnerable*, at risk of both self-neglect and exploitation by others. The law has long intervened in decision-making where the decision-maker is considered to lack mental capacity, either retrospectively (regarding past decisions) or prospectively (regarding future decisions). Certain legal principles (the principles of equity) will apply to evaluate retrospectively the decisions of the capable but vulnerable in the context of particular relationships – a personhood-centred approach embodied in legal doctrine. Those equitable principles, like the common law generally, originate in English law, and their interpretation by the English courts remains relevant to Canadian law.

The new question is whether and how far law's reach should extend prospectively where an individual cannot be said to lack mental capacity, but nevertheless appears unable to protect his or her best interests; a not uncommon situation for legal and health professionals interacting with older adults in general, and persons with dementia in particular. Answering this question requires a conceptual unpacking of the law that currently applies in this area, and a consideration of the underlying purpose and function of those existing legal rules. This chapter includes references to case law and, in places, details from certain cases to illustrate those rules and underlying principles.

DECISION-MAKING AND THE LAW

The vast run of human decision-making is, and remains, private, so far as the law is concerned; the law will not inquire into the prudence or foolishness, of private decisions. Risk can never be eliminated and, to the extent that risk is inherent in the idea of freedom, the elimination of risk has never been law's project. Law's ambit remains relatively narrow, and is always theoretically circumscribed; private decisions become publicly reviewable (through the operation of the law) only where justifiable for reasons of public policy.

The law intervenes to evaluate decisions and decision-making where the decision itself has legal implications or consequences (such as the contents of a will, the gift or sale of property, or the decision to marry) and where there are concerns relating to the decision-maker. Concerns relating to the decision-maker involve that person's perceived or alleged inability to understand and to protect his or her own best interests. Legal definitions and ideas of capacity and vulnerability are related to this concern. Decisions are subject to legal evaluation where both conditions are present – where the decision itself is inherently 'public' in that it has legal consequences, and where a legitimate protective role for the law has been recognized. Neither category is self-evident or closed; the categories of both decisions and decision-makers, which should be open to legal evaluation, are constantly contested and reviewed.

CAPACITY AND CONSENT

The common law evaluates decisions through two kinds of tests: tests related to the ability of a person to appreciate and understand (a quality referred to as 'capacity') and tests focusing on the individual's ability to give free or 'true' consent by reason of the context in which the decision is made.

Capacity

Legal capacity refers generally to an individual's internal or organic ability to make an informed choice with respect to a certain decision. Capacity may be evaluated or assessed retrospectively or prospectively. The purpose, and consequences, of retrospective and prospective evaluation are very different. Retrospective evaluation assesses capacity and/or consent at the time when past decisions were made; predictive evaluation assesses current and future capacity for decision-making. The purpose of retrospective evaluation is to determine whether past decisions were valid and should therefore be given legal effect. Predictive evaluation allows for intervention into ongoing, current situations and precedes appointment of a substitute decision-maker. In all cases incapacity is considered to flow from the individual's status or condition, as opposed to his or her situation or context.

Capacity is a *legal* concept – a determination made by a judge or master in a court of law, referring to medical evidence among other kinds of evidence. The mere presence of disease or infirmity will never in itself be sufficient to prove incapacity. Medical evidence is of course important and compelling but it is *evidence*, and not in itself conclusive, or even necessary in all instances unless required by statute (*Bridger* v. *Bridger* 2005 BCSC 269). Where any element of ambiguity exists, there is no objective medical test that will conclusively establish capacity.

Retrospective evaluation / assessment

The common law provides that a decision will be void where the decision-maker, at the relevant time, did not have the capacity required to make that particular decision. What must be considered in each case is the nature of the decision involved, and whether the necessary ability to make an informed choice about that decision was present. One may be capable of informed choice with regard to a relatively simple decision (such as marriage), while incapable of doing so with regard to a more complex decision (such as granting a power of attorney).

At first blush it appears striking that a decision with far-reaching and highly significant consequences for an individual's lifestyle and property (such as marriage) should require a low threshold of capacity that, once proven, places that decision beyond legal review (a private decision, however much regretted). The capacity threshold for marriage is relatively low because the subject matter – the pith of marriage that needs to be grasped, what marriage is about – is simple. A power of attorney, on the other hand, involves a relatively complex decision about legal arrangements dealing with financial and property matters and the capacity required of a donor is correspondingly higher. Note that both kinds of decisions are decisions with legal consequence; decisions without legal consequence (such as the decision to live together, without marriage) would generally be considered private and not reviewable (although where family-relations legislation treats co-habiting relationships as having legal consequences for the purposes of property division, it may be necessary to revaluate this public/private distinction).

The case of *Calvert* v. *Calvert* (1997), 32 OR (3d) 281 provides an interesting illustration of the common law approach to retrospective capacity assessment and, in particular, the 'degrees' of legal capacity. The case involved three different capacities, respecting decisions of different degrees of complexity and sophistication: the capacity to separate; the capacity to divorce; and the capacity to instruct counsel. Of these three, the decision to separate is the simplest and requires the lowest degree of capacity. The essence of the decision here is to know with whom one does not want to live. The decision to divorce is more complex than simply not living together; what is required is the desire to remain separate and no longer be married to one's spouse. The capacity to instruct counsel is significantly higher on the competency hierarchy as it involves the capacity to understand financial and legal issues.

The court determined that Mrs Calvert, in the early stages of Alzheimer's disease at the time the events in question took place, lacked capacity to instruct counsel. This did not mean, however, that she lacked the capacity to make personal decisions about where and with whom she wished to live. Indeed, the court referred to the underlying principle that the law will be especially careful to protect personal autonomy with regard to personal decisions of this kind. The court criticized a physician's testimony that Mrs Calvert's lack of explanation for why she had chosen to leave when she did, in light of her past expressed values against divorce, was evidence of her lack of capacity to separate. The true, underlying question was whether Mrs Calvert knew what she was doing, and the evidence showed that yes, clearly, she did. Once it was established that Mrs Calvert was capable of separating from her husband, her litigation guardian was able to pursue divorce on her behalf.

Although Mrs Calvert was not required to provide a rationale for her decision to leave her husband, the court provides her with an explanation that, poignantly and very humanly, takes her diminishing capacity into consideration – not as an impediment to her reasoning but, rather, as providing her with a reason to leave:

> The evidence is clear that she was...losing her cognitive abilities... The reaction of her husband and son-in-law to this was unsupportive... This, coupled with her long standing unhappiness with lack of funds, could have easily caused her to realise that, if she was going to leave, it had to be then... I believe she knew what the future held for her if she returned to Toronto... She feared being put out to pasture when her usefulness expired... She had been treated like a failure... I believe she viewed the progression of her life as intolerable... And she made one last, reasonable effort, before her abilities declined to the extent that she could not do so, to help herself.

The *Calvert* case, telling the story of a woman's lengthy, sometimes ambiguous, and non-linear decline into dementia, is also interesting as an illustration of the sometimes elusive nature and quality of capacity in the early stages of Alzheimer's disease. There is no sharp or obvious dividing line between 'capacity' and 'incapacity', as the subject moves between points of lucidity and confusion. Indeed, these points are not self-evident in themselves but, to a certain extent, are dependent on the observer. Numerous incidents are described which, according to Mrs Calvert's husband and son-in-law, clearly 'show' her mental deterioration; others, describing the same incidents, 'see' them as indicating something very different.

Predictive evaluation/assessment

The legal mechanism for a predictive finding of incapacity is found in legislation, not common law principle. The distinction between retrospective evaluation/assessment of capacity and prospective evaluation/assessment of capacity is significant. In the prospective process, the determination of incapacity goes not to a particular decision (as in the *Calvert* case), but to a more global class of decisions such as the ability to make decisions regarding one's person or one's estate. An individual who is found to be incapable of making these kinds of decision is protected from the consequences of his or her incapacity through the appointment of a substitute decision-maker (sometimes referred to as a 'guardian' or 'committee'). The consequence flowing from a finding that a person was not competent to make a particular past decision (granting a power of attorney, for example) is simply to set aside that particular transaction; no future consequences are necessarily implied. A finding that a person is incapable of managing his or her estate, in contrast, and the appointment of a committee of estate for that person, is all about future consequences. Previous decisions are not impugned, but the order affects, in a very dramatic sense, how all future decisions in this area will be made. Legislation (statutes, not common law principles) determines the mechanism for, and the circumstances in which, a finding of incapacity can be made for the purpose of appointing a substitute decision-maker.

A determination of incapacity preceding guardianship raises the most significant concerns about the relationship between the law relating to capacity and personal autonomy. It is important to bear in mind that this kind of determination is not the only kind of 'legal capacity', however, or the only context in which legal capacity is evaluated. A finding of legal capacity involving a particular past decision is an evaluation of a particular decision made at a particular time without necessary future implications (although factually a prospective finding of incapacity and appointment of a substitute decision-maker may follow a retrospective finding of incapacity, in a different proceeding). We don't hold a person responsible for the legal consequences of selling her house, for example, if she was not capable of making that decision at that time. The implications for personal autonomy in that kind of evaluation are present, but much less significant than where the evaluation limits future decision-making and imposes a substitute decision-maker.

Equity theory: Consent in situational context

Lack of capacity has an obvious impact on a person's ability to give consent; if I lack the mental capacity to appreciate and understand a decision, I obviously cannot be considered to have truly consented to it. The law also recognizes that consent may be vitiated in other ways, however, and for other reasons. The equitable doctrines of undue influence and unconscionability are explanations or theories for how the interaction between individual characteristics, social context and relationship context may work to impair a person's ability to consent truly or freely to a particular decision made in that context. Distinguished from incapacity, equity explains impaired consent with reference to the situation, or context, rather than the internally generated and fixed state of the individual (the *individual* is incapable; the *situation* is one of undue influence, or the transaction is unconscionable).

The characteristics of the individual will nevertheless be relevant to the analysis of impaired consent arising by reason of situation and not internal condition. Relevant characteristics include the declining/fluctuating mental processes of early dementia and increased isolation as the social connections formerly supplied by employment or parenting tend to fall away. Changes in physical health and/or ability that increase dependence or fearfulness may give rise to increased emotional vulnerability for many (although not necessarily all). Characteristics associated with the current generation of older adults may also work to increase vulnerability. Older adults are more likely to have a lower level of education, for example. The rapid technological and social changes of the last two decades may be confusing, particularly for women within the current generation of older adults who have spent their lives in traditional marriages without independent access to, or control of, economic resources.

None of these factors are, in themselves, sufficient to establish incapacity; they are perhaps best described as *sources of vulnerability*. When any of these or similar factors combine with a particular relationship power dynamic, the individual will be vulnerable to the 'undue' influence of or exploitation by another even though that individual is 'capable' (in the sense of having mental capacity) of making the decision. Indeed the subject of an undue influence or unconscionability analysis will always be 'capable' in this sense; if not, the case

would be decided on that lack of capacity and the decision set aside. Equity's vulnerability is distinct, by definition, from incapacity, and the connection to context and relationship situates the equitable analysis as a personhood-centred approach.

Undue influence

Birks and Chin (1997) describe undue influence as a 'plaintiff-sided' doctrine or theory; the focus of the inquiry is on the experience of the decision-maker and not the intentions, wicked or blameless, of the 'influencer'. Cases of undue influence may in fact involve intentional manipulation or exploitation: 'Give me the house or I'll make your life a misery', 'Give me $10,000 or I won't be able to help you anymore', 'Support me in your house or you'll never see your grandson again.'

In other kinds of situations, influence may become 'undue' not by reason of another's intentional pressure, but by reason of the power dynamics inherent in the relationship itself. Indeed, the good son who acts only in his mother's best interests, described by the court as 'honest, reliable, very reserved and anything but aggressive and demanding', may nevertheless exert undue influence over his mother through her 'confidence and trust' in him, justified though that may be (*Zed* v. *Zed* (1980), 28 NBR (2d) 580 (QB)). This quality of undue influence is described as 'presumed' undue influence; where there is a 'potential for domination inherent in the relationship itself' (*Geffen* v. *Goodman Estate*, [1991] 2 SCR 353) and where the 'weaker' party has conferred a benefit on the stronger, it is presumed that the benefit was the result of 'undue influence' arising from the relationship. In this kind of situation the responsibility is on the stronger party to displace that presumption, and to show affirmatively that in fact the consent, despite the relationship context, was freely given.

Some kinds of relationships will always give rise to a presumption of undue influence: doctor and patient, lawyer and client, for example. Other kinds of relationships must be examined on their particular facts to determine if they are of a kind and quality that will give rise to the presumption. There is no exact formula or measure for determining when influence will be 'undue' or for categorizing the kinds of relationship that may give rise to the presumption. 'It is neither feasible nor desirable to attempt too closely to define the relationship, or its characteristics, or the demarcation line showing the exact transition point where a relationship that does not entail the duty passes into one that does' (*Lloyds Bank* v. *Bundy*, [1974] 3 All ER 757 (CA)). The question depends on the particular facts of the case, and there is 'no substitute in this branch of the law for the meticulous examination of those facts' (*National Westminster Bank plc* v. *Morgan* (1985), 17 HLR 360).

The presumption may seem harsh where undue influence has not been exercised intentionally and, indeed, may have arisen through the blameless support and assistance provided by the 'stronger' person in the relationship to the dependent or 'weaker' one. This kind of helping relationship was found to give rise to a (non-displaced) presumption of undue influence in the case of *Gammon* v. *Steeves*, [1987] NBJ No. 1046 (NBCA), in which a niece and her husband had provided support and assistance to an elderly uncle and aunt. The aunt and uncle were both in ill health and had recently moved to the area, making them particularly dependent on the niece and her family. The older couple transferred property to the niece; following the death of his wife the uncle sought to have the transfer set aside. The court found that the relationship gave rise to a presumption of undue influence, although there was no evidence of the niece or her husband having coerced or intentionally pressured the uncle, noting in passing judgment: 'I come to this conclusion… reluctantly, as I am sure the trial judge did, because it is clear that Mr. and Mrs. Steeves spent considerable time and energy caring for Mr. and Mrs. Gammon at a time when no other relative was willing to do so. But this only points up the caution with which people must act when they accept gifts in these circumstances.' (See also *Love Estate* v. *Clements*, [1993] BCJ No. 2058 (SC); *Lowes* v. *Fitzgerald*, [1991] BCJ No. 3400 (SC); *Ogilvie* v. *Ogilvie Estate* (1998), 49 BCLR (3d) 277 (CA).) A helping relationship giving rise to a presumption of undue influence was also found in *Piscitelli* v. *Dinelle*, [1999] OJ No. 4396 (Ont. Ct. Jus.), [2001] OJ No. 1743 (Ont. CA), but in that case the presumption was rebutted successfully.

The policy rationale for the rule was described by Sir Erich Sachs in the case of *Lloyds Bank* v. *Bundy*: the court 'interferes not on the ground that any wrongful act has been committed by the donee but on the ground of public policy and to prevent the relations which existed between the parties and the influence arising from being abused'. Relationships giving rise to a presumption of undue influence are by their nature private and the 'dominant figure' in that relationship is the only one in a position to prevent that influence from being 'abused'. 'Abuse' in this context

> means no more than that once the existence of a special relationship has been established, then any possible use of the relevant influence is, irrespective of the intentions of the persons possessing it, regarded in relation to the transaction under consideration as an abuse – unless and until the duty of fiduciary care has been shown to be fulfilled or the transaction is shown to be truly for the benefit of the person influenced.

It is for this reason both fair and just to require that dominant figure, where he or she has received a benefit in the context of that relationship, to take active steps to ensure that the transaction was indeed freely chosen.

Personal characteristics associated with vulnerability will be relevant to the determination of whether a particular relationship will give rise to the presumption. In other words, part of the answer to the question of whether 'the potential for domination is inherent in the relationship itself' will turn on the personal characteristics of the 'weaker' party. If the potential for domination flows from dependence, an important source and feature of unintentional undue influence, individual characteristics going to dependency will be relevant (including emotional and psychological characteristics as well as physical). The presence of a dementia would undoubtedly lead to questions about undue influence. Relationship vulnerability is associated with personal vulnerability; it is possible to experience personal vulnerability without relationship vulnerability, but not vice versa.

Age is often treated as a relevant factor, for both objective reasons relating to physical or mental decline, or increased physical dependence, and subjective reasons relating to emotional pressures and family dynamics. *Stel-Van Homes Ltd.* v. *Fortini* (2001), 16 BLR (3d) 103 (Ont. SCJ) explains how the desire to keep the family peace can make older family members vulnerable to pressures. The plaintiff in that case was an older father of grown children who had emigrated from Italy to Canada many years before, subsequently building up a successful construction company. One of his sons-in-law began to pursue the plaintiff to hand over his shares in the company to 'the boys' (another son-in-law was prepared to go along with whatever the plaintiff decided). The plaintiff, aware of his increasing age and experiencing health difficulties, had wanted to scale down his involvement with the company, but did not wish to withdraw altogether. The son-in-law and his wife, the plaintiff's daughter, were experiencing marital difficulties during this period, making the plaintiff more anxious to keep the peace in the interests of his daughter's marriage. Choosing the interests of family harmony over his own interests, the plaintiff agreed to transfer the shares. The plaintiff agreed to the transfer; soon afterwards, his daughter's marriage came to an end. The court found that the pressure exerted on the plaintiff by the defendant son-in-law through his persistent badgering about the transfer, in the context of the plaintiff's position within the wider network of family relationships, amounted to intentional undue influence and that the relationship gave rise to an (un-rebutted) presumption of undue influence.

Lord Browne-Wilkinson, in *Barclays Bank* v. *O'Brien*, [1994] 1 AC 180 (HL), concluded that the relationship between 'aged parents' and adult children should be treated as one of several intimate relationships in which the question of whether the presumption arises should be treated by the courts with a 'special tenderness', referring to the case of *Avon* v. *Bridger*, [1985] 2 All ER 281 (CA), involving older parents and adult children. The 'special tenderness' class was defined with reference to the emotional and psychological ties inherent in certain relationships of intimacy, including relationships of co-habitation. Those factors make it more likely that a presumption of undue influence would be justified. Informal transactions, without professional input, would also be more likely in the context of intimate relationships.

Inter-generational relationships involving help or care will not give rise to the presumption of undue influence in every circumstance; *Calumsky* v. *Karaloff*, [1946] SCR 110, *Kits Estate* v. *Peterson* (1994), 161 AR 299 (QB), *Zabolotney Estate Committee* v. *Szyjak* (1980), 5 Man. R. (2d) 107 (QB), *Scott* v. *Clancy*, [1998] WWR 446 (Sask. QB), and *Tracy* v. *Boles*, [1996] BCJ No. 52 (SC) are all cases in which an older transferor trusted, was grateful to and in some respects depended on the transferee but where the younger person was not the dominant figure in the relationship. In all of these cases, the personal characteristics of the older person were significant; an older person with some physical dependence may nevertheless be psychologically independent, even the dominating party in the relationship. The narrative provided in the cases of *Re Brocklehurst*, [1978] 1 All ER 767 (CA) and *Shortell* v. *Fitzpatrick*, [1949] OR 488 provide detailed and subtle (and, in *Re Brocklehurst*, contested) accounts of this kind of relationship.

The doctrine of undue influence (like unconscionability, discussed below) describes a source and quality of vulnerability, and its effect on decision-making, separate and apart from the idea of capacity. The doctrines in effect stake out a set of circumstances in which the law will intervene in decision-making on the basis of the individual's situational vulnerability. Explaining that vulnerability in terms of the interaction between the individual and his or her context, including relationship context, equity's theoretical framework allows us to 'see' vulnerability outside of incapacity as legally relevant. This focus on the whole individual, including the personal variability it provides for, shares important characteristics with the personhood approach.

Unconscionability

The distinction between unconscionability and undue influence was explained in the Australian case of *Commercial Bank of Australia* v. *Amadio* (1983), 151 CLR 461 as a distinction between exploitation, on the one hand, and impaired consent, on the other:

In the latter [undue influence] the will of the innocent party is not independent and voluntary because it is overborne. In the former [unconscionability] the will of the innocent party, even if independent and voluntary, is the result of the disadvantageous position in which he or she is placed and out of the other party's unconscientiously taking advantage of that position.

Equity sets aside transactions that are deemed to be 'unconscionable' on the basis of exploitation; it would be inequitable to give the unconscionable transaction legal effect because it is the product of one person's exploitation of another. If undue influence is 'plaintiff-sided', unconscionability is a 'defendant-sided' doctrine; the inequity arises from the conduct of the defendant. There can be no unintentional unconscionability.

Unconscionability, like undue influence, is about vulnerability that is both constructed and situational as opposed to internal and organic. Where an inequality between the parties ('inequality' defined with reference to the power balance of the relationship in question) puts one (the 'weaker') in the power of the other (the 'stronger'), and where the bargain is substantially unfair to the benefit of the stronger, a presumption of unconscionability will be raised. This presumption will be rebutted if the defendant can show that the bargain was fair, just and reasonable.

Inequality in this context refers not to objective inequalities such as physical disabilities, but to an inequality that, in the context of the relationship, impairs the individual's ability to protect his or her own best interests. A blind person, for example, may well be capable of protecting his or her interests and, if so, will not be 'weaker' in the sense that he or she is in the power of the other player in the relationship (see, for example, *Sperling Estate* v. *Heidt* (1998), 178 Sask. R. 192 (QB), aff'd. (2000), 199 Sask. R. 256 (CA)). Chronic drunkenness, in comparison, is more likely to have the relevant psychological effect, striking at the ability of an individual to advance or protect his interests. The defendant who knowingly takes advantage of that inability will be behaving unconscionably for the purposes of the doctrine (see *Black* v. *Wilcox* (1976), 12 OR (2d) 759 (CA)).

Age, like other objective 'weakness', does not in itself create an inequality for the purposes of unconscionability. Nor should age itself be an independent factor going to the balance of power between the parties. Many factors or characteristics generally associated with the ageing process will be relevant in this context, however: loneliness and social dependence; fearfulness about the future (who will provide for me if not the 'stronger' party?); a lack of knowledge regarding current business practices and values; the lack of assertiveness and confidence that may accompany physical decline; the occa-sional confusion and lack of clarity of early-stage dementia. What must be shown, where the relevant weakness exists, is that the stronger party took advantage of that weakness to the detriment of the weaker.

Hall and Hall v. *Grassie Estate*, [1982] MJ No. 339, 16 Man. R. (2d) 399 (QB) provides an example of circumstances in which a transaction was set aside as unconscionable. The transferor in that case, Mrs Grassie, was an 85-year-old woman who was described as 'regularly in a confused state', and her 'capacity to decide anything…very limited at best' (there was no finding of incapacity, however). Her physical health was poor. Prior to moving into a nursing home Mrs Grassie had lived in the same house (the subject of the transfer) since the 1920s and had no understanding of contemporary real estate prices. The defendants, long-time acquaintances of Mrs Grassie, were described as 'much younger, healthy, active and experienced in real estate transactions'. The purchase price was much lower than the actual value of the house, as the defen-dants must have appreciated.

The court concluded that the situation 'cried out for independent advice' which Mrs Grassie did not receive. The defendants' own lawyer had acted for both parties in the sale. Given her personal circumstances, Mrs Grassie was unable to protect her own best interests and the circumstances indicated that the defendants understood this and sought to take advantage of the older woman's relative weakness. The transaction was set aside as unconscionable.

The case of *Matheson Estate* v. *Stefankiw* (2001), 191 Sask. R. 241 (QB) also involved an older adult who appears to have been in the earlier stages of cognitive decline, and a transfer of property for less than market value. In this case however, unlike *Grassie*, the court found that the transfer was not uncon-scionable. The elderly transferee, Matheson (now deceased), had transferred farmland at a price below its actual value. The transferors were long-term tenants on the farmland in question. Mr Matheson showed several signs of objective weakness: he had become increasingly reclusive and fearful of dealing with strangers. His health and hygiene had deteriorated to a striking degree. He had begun to experience occasional delusional episodes – not suffi-cient, apparently, to lead to a conclusion of incapacity but sufficient to place Mr Matheson in the 'grey zone'. The tenants had provided assistance to Mr Matheson over the years, and he was comfortable with them.

The court concluded that, in the circumstances, Mr Matheson had obtained something of real value aside from the price paid for his property. Mr Mathe-son's gratitude to his tenants, and ability to express his gratitude through the transfer, had worth to him. The transfer to his tenants had also spared him the 'agony' of having to deal with strangers. The tenants had not initiated the transfer – it was Mr Matheson's idea – nor was there any evidence that they had pursued the transfer or in any other way sought to exploit their neighbour and landlord. Aware of Mr Matheson's increasing difficulties, the tenants responded with assistance and support, rather than exploitation. Under the circumstances, the transaction was not unconscionable.

Matheson and *Grassie* illustrate the contextual analysis of vulnerability within the doctrine of unconscionability. Mere age, even age together with evidence of cognitive decline, does not equate to vulnerability for the purposes of either the unconscionability or undue influence analysis. The focus is on the interaction between individual vulnerability, social vulnerability and relationship vulnerability – where that interaction creates a heightened vulnerability or risk of unfairness, the law will intervene to evaluate a decision made in that context. Both undue influence and unconscionability provide an explicitly legal model for a personhood-centred evaluation of decision-making.

CONCLUSION: CAPACITY, CONSENT AND PERSONHOOD IN DECISION-MAKING

Individuals in early-stage dementia are not, necessarily or by definition, incapable of decision-making per se, although an individual may be incapable of making certain complex decisions. Personal characteristics associated with early-stage dementia will, in particular contexts, give rise to personal vulnerability justifying law's interest, evaluation and even intervention where that vulnerability is a source of harm and loss. Undue influence and unconscionability provide a sophisticated and tested legal theoretical framework for understanding that quality of situation-specific and personhood-centred vulnerability, and the legal significance of personhood in the evaluation of decision-making.

Traditional theories of undue influence and unconscionability apply to undo prior transactions, a retrospective evaluation. Policy makers are now grappling with the question of how, whether and when prospective evaluation and intervention (if not substitute decision-making) can be justified on the basis of vulnerability and its impact on decision-making, as opposed to lack of capacity. Equity's personhood-centred theories of vulnerability and its relationship to decision-making are essential to that discussion.

ACKNOWLEDGMENT

This work was supported in part through a Social Sciences and Humanities Research Foundation (SSHRC) Development Research Grant (#820-2006-1030).

REFERENCE

Birks, P. and Chin, N.Y. (1997) 'On the Nature of Undue Influence.' In J. Beatson and D. Friedman (eds) *Good Faith and Fault in Contract Law*. London: Clarendon Press.

CASES

Avon v. *Bridger*, [1985] 2 All ER 281 (CA)

Barclays Bank v. *O'Brien*, [1994] 1 AC 180 (HL)

Black v. *Wilcox* (1976), 12 OR (2d) 759 (CA)

Bridger v. *Bridger* 2005 BCSC 269

Re Brocklehurst, [1978] 1 All ER 767 (CA)

Calumsky v. *Karaloff*, [1946] SCR 110

Calvert v. *Calvert* (1997), 32 OR (3d) 281

Commercial Bank of Australia v. *Amadio* (1983), 151 CLR 461

Gammon v. *Steeves*, [1987] NBJ No. 1046 (NBCA)

Geffen v. *Goodman Estate*, [1991] 2 SCR 353

Hall and Hall v. *Grassie Estate*, [1982] MJ No. 339, 16 Man. R. (2d) 399 (QB)

Kits Estate v. *Peterson* (1994), 161 AR 299 (QB)

Lloyds Bank v. *Bundy*, [1974] 3 All ER 757 (CA)

Love Estate v. *Clements*, [1993] BCJ No. 2058 (SC)

Lowes v. *Fitzgerald*, [1991] BCJ No. 3400 (SC)

Matheson Estate v. *Stefankiw* (2001), 191 Sask. R. 241 (QB)

National Westminster Bank plc v. *Morgan* (1985), 17 HLR 360

Ogilvie v. *Ogilvie Estate* (1998), 49 BCLR (3d) 277 (CA)

Piscitelli v. *Dinelle*, [1999] OJ No. 4396 (Ont. Ct. Jus.), [2001] OJ No. 1743 (Ont. CA)

Scott v. *Clancy*, [1998] WWR 446 (Sask. QB)

Shortell v. *Fitzpatrick*, [1949] OR 488

Sperling Estate v. *Heidt* (1998), 178 Sask. R. 192 (QB), aff'd. (2000), 199 Sask. R. 256 (CA)

Stel-Van Homes Ltd. v. *Fortini* (2001), 16 BLR (3d) 103 (Ont. SCJ)

Tracy v. *Boles*, [1996] BCJ No. 52 (SC)

Zabolotney Estate Committee v. *Szyjak* (1980), 5 Man. R. (2d) 107 (QB)

Zed v. *Zed* (1980), 28 NBR (2d) 580 (QB)

CHAPTER 10

Personhood, Financial Decision-Making and Dementia

An Australian Perspective

CHERYL TILSE, JILL WILSON AND DEBORAH SETTERLUND

Personhood approaches to dementia care (Kitwood 1997) challenge the belief that people with dementia undergo a complete loss of self. In policy and practice, this means recognizing and supporting the ongoing abilities of people with dementia to make or participate in decisions about their lives (Wilkinson 2001). This chapter focuses on financial decision-making as a key area where older people with dementia can be included or excluded from decision-making. First, it briefly outlines the burgeoning interest in older people's financial assets as a context in which a range of protective responses is promoted. It then uses the findings from an Australian research program exploring asset management to examine the opportunities for and constraints on promoting a personhood approach to involving people with dementia in decision-making about their finances.

BACKGROUND

In societies with ageing populations, family, government and market interests in the management of older people's financial assets stem from a range of intersecting factors: recognition of the importance of assets to older people; competing interests in their use; enhanced emphasis on planning for later life; and the importance of assisted decision-making around financial matters. Each of these areas is briefly considered to outline the context of this practice area.

Assets have meaning socially, emotionally and culturally, as well as in economic terms. In many Western cultures, access to money and property is a key symbol of adult status and a power base from which to negotiate exchanges within social and economic systems. Langan and Means (1996) have argued that the importance of money and control over money for older people should not be underestimated. Studies of the gendered distribution of domestic monies in households have linked access to money with questions of equality, power and control (Singh 1996; Zelizer 1995). At a practical level, assets are core to older people's well-being in retaining choices in housing, care and lifestyle options. Consideration thus needs to be given to the social, cultural and psychological meanings of money in the processes and practices surrounding determinations of capacity to make or be involved in financial decisions.

Asset management can be an area of complicated decision-making as a result of competing interests in older people's assets and the complexity of retirement incomes. Older people's preferences in the use of their assets can compete with those of family members who may seek to protect an inheritance, and with state and service providers seeking to enhance user contributions to the costs of care (Tilse, Wilson et al. 2005). In addition, asset management can require complex decision-making when combinations of occupational, state or overseas pensions, property and investments need to be prudently managed over an extended period of time. In later life, opportunities to generate or regenerate an asset base are reduced. Mistakes in asset management are thus likely to have long-term implications for future care and lifestyle choices.

Policy concerns about the increasing proportions of older people with dementia have fostered an emphasis on later life planning, assessment of capacity and substitute decision-making. In addition, emerging concerns about financial elder abuse have promoted interest in protective responses (Rabiner, O'Keeffe and Brown 2004). Wilbur (2001) highlights the related problems of doing too much or too little for adults with diminished decision-making capacity. She notes that the legal substitute decision-making mechanisms are fairly blunt instruments that are more likely to foster doing too much. A core concern in developing legislative responses to elder abuse is how to balance empowerment and protection (Doron, Alon and Offir 2004).

A diagnosis of dementia generally raises, very early, concerns about capacity to make financial decisions and the need to protect financial assets. A diagnosis of dementia, however, does not and should not automatically mean a judgement of incapacity to make decisions (Horton-Deutsch and Evans 2007; Marson 2002; Tyrrell, Genin and Myslinski 2006). Despite extensive studies on capacity assessment, the day-to-day issues of the decision-making process and the ways people with dementia can be supported to remain involved are not well understood (Horton-Deutsch and Evans 2007; Tyrrell *et al.* 2006). In 2002, Marson anticipated that future research will involve 'interventional studies that seek to support decisional autonomy of older adults in areas such as consenting to medical treatment, consenting to participate in research, and managing financial affairs' (p.101).

Currently, little is known about the nature of the involvement of people with dementia in financial decision-making and how participation might be achieved in ways that empower older people, protect assets and not impose extensive tasks on carers. In order to provide insights into the opportunities and constraints within formal and informal financial decision-making, the Assets and Ageing research program at the University of Queensland, Australia (Tilse, Wilson *et al.* 2007), aims to explore, describe and explain current practices of non-professional asset management from the perspectives of informal carers, older people and care providers. The research program seeks to raise awareness of this little-understood area of care and to identify practices that combine empowerment with protection for both older people and their families. It also aims to recognize and support the role of families/informal carers in making day-to-day assessments of capacity to engage in financial decision-making. Within the program, asset management is conceptualized as having some control over organizing, decision-making and/or use of an older person's economic assets. Both income and capital assets are included.

The program comprises a series of linked research projects. This chapter uses findings from four research projects. These are: a national prevalence study of the involvement of family, friends and neighbours in asset management for and with older people (Tilse, Setterlund *et al.* 2005); an in-depth study of the practices and preferences of family carers managing assets for and with older people (Tilse, Wilson *et al.* 2005); an in-depth study of the preferences and experiences of older people in receipt of asset management assistance (Tilse, Setterlund *et al.* 2007); and a study of the factors contributing to the financial abuse of older people with impaired capacity (McCawley *et al.* 2006).

FINANCIAL DECISION-MAKING AND DEMENTIA

Paying bills, managing paperwork and making decisions about money, property and investments are tasks that require memory, reasoning and comprehension, a capacity to define situations and to hold a task in sequence. Dementia can affect all of these abilities. The capacity to self-manage some or all of such tasks is therefore likely to be questioned by older people, family members or carers, and appropriate formal or informal assistance may be sought.

Formal responses to financial decision-making

In many countries, substitute decision-making legislation seeks to address limitations in the capacity of people to make financial, person and/or healthcare decisions. Substitute decision-making legislation in relation to financial matters (commonly called enduring or durable powers of attorney or financial guardianship) provides a legal authority for others to make financial decisions for older people who are assessed as having impairments in decision-making capacity. Emerging critiques of such legislation have questioned whether the formal instrument has facilitated financial abuse rather than protected older people's assets, and whether a balance between empowerment and protection has been achieved (McCawley *et al.* 2006; Wilbur 2001).

Assessment of capacity to make decisions is central to substitute decision-making legislation. In understanding capacity, many jurisdictions have moved from a status approach, which views a person with impairment as having a global decision-making incapacity, to a decision-specific and situational approach, in which capacity is considered in relation to a specific decision at a specific time and under specific circumstances (e.g. the UK Mental Capacity Act 2005 – see Department for Consitutional Affairs (UK) 2007, p.19). This approach recognizes that capacity depends on the interaction between a person's impairment and their circumstances. It promotes the provision of information and support to a person to enhance their capacity to make a particular decision and, in some jurisdictions, to communicate that decision rather than make the decision for them. It begins with a presumption of capacity.

In Queensland, Australia, the Guardianship and Administration Act 2000 defines capacity in a decision-specific manner, provides for the presumption of capacity, and recognizes that capacity to make decisions may differ according to the nature and extent of the impairment, the type of decision to be made, and the support available from members of the adult's existing network. The legislation is underpinned by a 'least restrictive alternative' approach, promoting assisted decision-making as well as substituted decision-making. This reflects a concern with balancing empowerment and protection. Despite this, when issues of decision-making capacity are raised, the emphasis in practice has generally been on taking over decision-making (substituted decision-making) and protecting older people from financial abuse rather than on developing strategies and techniques to assist older people to retain some degree of involvement in managing their assets.

The moral, ethical and social, as well as the clinical, dimensions of capacity or competency assessments are increasingly recognized. Marson (2002) citing Grisso (1986) proposes that 'competency judgements are ultimately moral judgements insofar as the clinician or judge acts as a proxy for society in determining whether an individual should retain autonomy in a set of activities' (p.101). The importance of assets to well-being, competing interests in older people's assets, concerns about financial abuse and the socio-cultural value placed on money can promote approaches that limit risk, are overly protective and move to substituted decision-making as a first option rather than exploring assisted decision-making. Advice to engage in advanced planning as soon as possible after a diagnosis of dementia is generally taken up in the area of financial matters especially in relation to enduring powers of attorney and wills (Cohen 2004). Although this is important and timely advice, these approaches can lead some to equate dementia with incapacity and obscure the remaining capacities.

Informal involvement in financial decision-making

Assistance with managing assets is most commonly provided by family members and, to a lesser extent, friends and neighbours (Tilse, Setterlund *et al.* 2005). Assistance is provided for a range of reasons – lack of confidence, sensory and mobility problems, frailty and dementia – not all of which are related to a decision-making incapacity. This suggests that there are structural and attitudinal barriers as well as issues of cognitive impairment that limit older people's involvement in this area (Tilse, Setterlund *et al.* 2005). These contextual barriers may well be magnified when there is a diagnosis of dementia.

Families assist with the everyday tasks of banking and paying bills and more complex tasks of managing investments and property. They use formal (e.g. enduring power of attorney arrangements), semi-formal (e.g. bank or nominee arrangements) and informal mechanisms (e.g. using personal identification numbers to access bank accounts) to assist older people (Tilse, Setterlund *et al.* 2005). Any of these practices can be used in a well-considered, risky or abusive manner. Any of these practices can include or exclude the older person in decision-making.

In the in-depth study of asset managers (Tilse, Wilson *et al.* 2005), acting to include the older person in decision-making rather than simply taking over as a substitute decision-maker is reported to be time-consuming and difficult.

Carers identified particular difficulties in relation to assisting an older person with dementia. These difficulties were: the time taken to involve the older person in decisions; communicating decisions and complex information; and in making decisions for others when current or past preferences were not clearly known or articulated.

Some participants reported practices that are risky for the older person and/or the carer. These practices included limited record-keeping, mingling family accounts with those of the older person, and paying with their own money and then reimbursing themselves through access to the older person's accounts. Such practices often arose from issues of convenience for the asset manager, a sense of trust in families or a limited awareness of accountability responsibilities of an asset manager. Some carers and older people also described practices that excluded and disempowered older people through ageist, sexist and disablist assumptions, or through family attitudes of entitlement to older people's money and property.

The study of asset managers and an analysis of the files of older people with impaired capacity coming to the attention of the Guardianship and Administrative Tribunal of Queensland (McCawley *et al.* 2006) also found that some carers openly acknowledged that they had misappropriated the assets of older people. In the carer study (Tilse, Wilson *et al.* 2005) such disclosures were freely made by some participants in response to questions about their practices in managing the assets of older people. This group generally did not see that their behaviour was problematic – there was a sense of entitlement underpinned by the belief that the older person would not 'mind' or 'didn't need it anymore'. In the file audit 26 per cent of cases were classified as reflecting abusive behaviour, with 77 per cent of these cases involving the deliberate stripping of older people's assets, and the remainder inappropriately using older people's assets through ignorance, or the failing capacity of the carer. Such abuse is more likely to occur when the carer has unmonitored, legally authorized access to the older person's assets.

The personhood literature (Jaworksa 1997; Kitwood 1999) proposes that older people with dementia are undervalued as people. The findings from the Assets and Ageing research program also suggest that prevailing attitudes to older people who require assistance with managing their assets allow some people to think that it is acceptable to 'help yourself' to their assets even though this can result in a severe detriment to the older person. These sets of assumptions can be a serious barrier to promoting the inclusion of older people with dementia in some decision-making about their financial affairs.

OLDER PEOPLE'S PREFERENCES

The in-depth study exploring older people's experiences of having their assets managed (Tilse, Setterlund *et al.* 2007) did not focus specifically on older people with dementia. The issues raised in relation to inclusive asset management practice, however, provide a base from which to explore how to retain the personhood of the older person with dementia when making financial decisions for and with them. In seeking to understand how protection and empowerment are balanced in current practices, the research uses the conceptualization of Secker *et al.* (2003) in the United Kingdom. These authors have argued for an understanding of independence that takes account of two intersecting dimensions: reliance on others for assistance and the subjective experience of receiving help. Independence is high when an older person's experience of receiving assistance matches their 'desired level of choice, social usefulness and autonomy' (Secker *et al.* 2003, p.381). The Australian research was interested in the level and form of participation older people retain when receiving asset management help, whether this was congruent with their wishes and what factors facilitate or prevent continuing participation (Tilse, Setterlund *et al.* 2007).

The analysis of the in-depth interviews identified three asset management scenarios. The scenarios, reported elsewhere (Tilse, Setterlund *et al.* 2007), highlight the importance of recognizing that the desired level of involvement in asset management varies between older people and for each older person in different contexts or at different times. Older people's preferences ranged from full participation and control over decision-making with others implementing the decisions, partial participation through monitoring or consultation about decisions, to no participation stemming either from a desire to hand over tasks to others or from a family member's unwillingness to involve the older person in decisions. Older people identified the importance of managing within the context of family relationships, a common response being a desire to prioritize maintaining relationships over the quality of asset management being provided.

Empowering practices are characterized by a high level of congruence between the needs and expectations of older people and the practical and emotional capacity of their carers to meet those expectations. Responses to older people are more likely to be empowering when the older person's rights in relation to their assets are not contested and the carer has the resources to respond flexibly to the older person's needs. The next section identifies some core practice principles for person-centred practice.

IMPLICATIONS FOR PERSON-CENTRED PRACTICE

The research program demonstrates that decision-making in relation to asset management takes place in a social, cultural, legal, ethical, family and financial context. Developing and supporting person-centred practice in this arena will need to consider all of these domains and attend to the interface between the individual and her/his interpersonal and socio-cultural environment.

Baldwin (2008; see also this volume) asserts that personhood requires agency and opportunity. A key challenge for policy, legislation and practice in financial decision-making is to understand how to recognize, promote and support agency, and provide opportunity. Further recognition of the environmental, attitudinal and legislative barriers to assisted decision-making will help in identifying opportunities to engage and support people with dementia at the level they desire and can manage. Person-centred practice will promote assisted, rather than substitute, decision-making as a first option. It is facilitated by a careful understanding of the experiences and desires of an older person in a particular context, a set of attitudes that focus on the value of the older person rather than the issues they live with, and sufficient resources to provide the most appropriate support for the older person. In financial decision-making we need to learn more about how to make decisions *with* rather than *for* people with dementia.

A personhood focus provides an important set of interrelated principles for developing a range of policy and practice responses that balance protection and empowerment around financial management for and with older people with dementia. This section outlines three of these principles: individualizing; balancing care and control; and recognizing that competence is fluid and varies with the nature of the task.

First, an individualizing rather than a global response is a fundamental principle for respecting the personhood of an older person in situations where decisional competence is challenged. In financial decision-making, an individual response is based on an understanding of the following: the nature of the task and the decision to be made; the capacity of the person to participate in that decision; the nature of that participation; and the preferences of the older person. A contextual/situational approach will add to this an understanding of the social, cultural, financial and family situation, the risks and implications of the financial decision, the carer's skills and preferences, the support available in existing networks, and the nature of the relationships that will be supported or challenged by asset management practices.

Second, day-to-day informal appraisals of capacity are made in the context of a relationship and the task under consideration. The tasks of financial management vary in their complexity and in the inherent longer-term risk to the older person's quality of life. Some are straightforward, others are highly complex requiring specialized knowledge or high-level skills. Decisions about competency thus vary as they are made in the context of day-to-day judgements relating to the particular decisions to be made or tasks to be completed in the context of understanding the personality of the older person. A response respecting personhood will view decision-making as a collaborative process and consider what the person values (Jaworska 1999). It might be carrying a wallet or purse with money in it, being able to purchase a cup of coffee, being consulted about how bills are being paid or being reassured that assets are being managed by trusted people.

Third, there is a growing recognition that decisional competence is not all or nothing but is spread across a wide continuum (Holm 2001), that some context-dependent decision-making abilities remain (Wilkinson 2001) and that practitioners must strive to identify and respect areas of competence. Some older people in early-stage dementia are likely to have some ability to manage, monitor or participate in some financial decision-making or tasks; others will be in need of assistance although this may vary with the complexity of the task or the decision. For some older people with dementia, involvement is likely to be limited. In addition, asset management assistance will be fraught with difficulty when there is paranoia that can be associated with some dementia.

An approach respecting personhood will make day-to-day judgements with the older person about what matters to them and what is the level of involvement possible and desired. For an older person, participation in asset management can vary from full control over decision-making to a sense of being consulted or at least being informed. A person-centred approach following Kitwood (1997) will focus on supporting the abilities a person has, enabling choice, providing comfort from anxiety (e.g. by knowing there is access to records or opportunity for discussion of asset management activities) and acknowledging the emotional responses linked to assets (e.g. expressing feelings of concern about whether there is sufficient money to provide for ongoing care). Older people will vary in their interest in remaining involved in asset management. Some will actively choose to remain involved, some will cede responsibilities to others, and others will prioritize sustaining family relationships over financial considerations.

The way an asset manager operates as a substitute or assisted decision-maker is thus likely to be dynamic – changing with changing situations and different times. This is a demanding task for carers, which is likely to require day-to-day judgements, support for the older person, and financial accountability as a prudent asset manager.

There are cultural values about managing money in families, and these values and the dynamics of the family will affect practices and perspectives on the opportunities that should be provided to the older person to remain involved. In addition, carers will vary in their ability and willingness to respond to the demands of including older people in decision-making. The nature of the asset management arrangement (e.g. whether the carer is a sole manager or has others to assist in managing assets), the complexity of the tasks, the formal and informal mechanisms in use, the understanding of accountability require-ments, the carer's experiences of the demands and rewards of being involved in care, anticipated inheritances, other demands on the carer's time and attention, and the quality of the relationship between the asset manager and the older person will all influence the approach taken to asset management decision-making.

CONCLUSION

Person-centred practice in managing assets is characterized by achieving a con-gruence between the task or decisions to be made, the older person's capacity to complete the task or participate in decision-making, her/his desire to be involved and the opportunities presented to participate. A key issue then is to describe and understand how greater participation in asset management can be nurtured and sustained for older people with dementia. Facilitating such practice will involve understanding the everyday practices that empower and include older people with dementia in their asset management to the extent that they desire and can manage, making sure carers are supported, and ensuring older people's assets are protected from misuse and abuse. In dementia care, this will require a commitment to core principles and skills in assessing, understanding and responding to individual, interactional and socio-cultural contexts.

REFERENCES

Baldwin, C. (2008) 'Narrative, citizenship and dementia: The personal and the political.' *Journal of Aging Studies 22,* 222–228.

Cohen, C. (2004) 'Surrogate decision making: Special issues in geriatric psychiatry.' *Canadian Journal of Psychiatry 47,* 7, 454–457.

Department for Constitutional Affairs (UK) (2007) *Mental Capacity Act 2005: Code of Practice* Available at www.opsi.gov.uk/ACTS/acts2005/related/ukpgacop_20050009_en.pdf, accessed 12 December 2008.

Doron, I., Alon, S. and Offir, N. (2004) 'Time for policy: Legislative response to elder abuse and neglect in Israel.' *Journal of Elder Abuse and Neglect 16,* 4, 63–82.

Grisso, T. (1986) *Evaluating Competencies: Forensic Assents and Instruments.* New York: Plenum Press.

Holm, S. (2001) 'Autonomy, authenticity, or best interest: Everyday decision-making and persons with dementia.' *Medicine, Health Care and Philosophy 4,* 153–159.

Horton-Deutsch, P.T. and Evans, R. (2007) 'Health care decision-making of persons with dementia.' *Dementia 6,* 1, 105–120.

Jaworska, A. (1999) 'Respecting the margins of agency: Alzheimer's patients and the capacity to value.' *Philosophy and Public Affairs 28,* 105–138.

Kitwood, T. (1997) *Dementia Reconsidered: The Person Comes First.* Buckingham: Open University Press.

Langan, J. and Means, R. (1996) 'Financial management and elderly people with dementia in the UK: As much as question of confusion as abuse?' *Ageing and Society 16,* 257–314.

Marson, D. (2002) 'Competency assessment and research in an aging society.' *Generations 26,* 1, 99–103.

McCawley, A., Tilse, C., Wilson, J., Setterlund, D. and Rosenman, L. (2006) 'Older people with impaired capacity and financial abuse.' *Journal of Adult Protection 8,* 1, 20–33.

Rabiner, D.J., O'Keeffe, J. and Brown, D. (2004) 'A conceptual framework of financial exploitation of older persons.' *Journal of Elder Abuse and Neglect 16,* 2, 53–73.

Secker, J., Hill, R., Villeneau, L. and Parkman, S. (2003) 'Promoting independence: But promoting what and how?' *Ageing and Society 23,* 375–391.

Singh, S. (1996) 'Money in heterosexual relationships.' *Journal of Sociology 32,* 3, 57–69.

Tilse, C., Setterlund, D., Wilson, J. and. Rosenman, L. (2005) 'Minding the money: A growing responsibility for informal carers.' *Ageing and Society 25,* 2, 215–227.

Tilse, C., Setterlund, D., Wilson, J. and Rosenman, L. (2007) 'Managing the financial assets of older people: Balancing independence and protection.' *British Journal of Social Work 37,* 565–572.

Tilse, C., Wilson, J., Setterlund, D. and Rosenman, L. (2005) 'Older people's assets: A contested site' *Australasian Journal on Ageing 24,* S1, S51–S56.

Tilse, C., Wilson, J., Setterlund, D. and Rosenman, L. (2007) 'The new caring: Financial management and older people.' *Annals of the New York Academy of Science 114,* 355–361.

Tyrrell, J., Genin, N. and Myslinski, M. (2006) 'Freedom of choice and decision-making in health and social care.' *Dementia 5,* 4, 479–501.

Wilbur, K. (2001) 'Decision-making, dementia and the law: Cross national perspectives.' *Aging and Mental Health 5,* 4, 309–311.

Wilkinson, H. (2001) 'Empowerment and decision making for people with dementia: The use of legal interventions in Scotland.' *Aging and Mental Health 5,* 4, 322–328.

Zelizer, V. (1995) *The Social Meaning of Money: Pin Money, Paychecks, Poor Relief, and Other Currencies.* New York: Basic Books.

PART 3

Understanding at the Everyday Level

CHAPTER 11

Analysing Decision-Making
Bridging and Balancing

JOHN KEADY, SION WILLIAMS AND JOHN
HUGHES-ROBERTS

OVERVIEW

The aim of this chapter is to introduce the concept of 'bridging' as a metaphor
and conceptual description for ongoing adaptation and decision-making
processes made by people living with Alzheimer's disease (AD), and their
support networks, throughout their experience of living with the condition.
Bridging was located within three sequential and transitional stages of living
with dementia: Losing Balance→Finding Balance→Keeping Balance.
Bridging was also seen to operate at two levels – 'strong' and 'weak' – with the
conditions surrounding each impacting upon day-to-day decision-making and
personal autonomy.

INTRODUCTION

As the literature reveals, a decision to seek and establish a diagnosis is one of the
most significant events in the experience of dementia, as it marks a status
passage between pre- and post-illness identity (Pratt and Wilkinson 2001).
Certainly, in the United Kingdom, the weight of social, practice and public
policy recommendations are stridently in favour of early diagnosis (Care
Services Improvement Partnership 2005; Department of Health 2001;
National Institute for Health and Clinical Excellence/Social Care Institute for
Excellence 2006), and this outcome forms an integral component of the
Dementia Strategy in England (Banerjee and Chan 2008; Department of

Health 2008). However, whilst this remains a central policy and service goal, it must be remembered that the early manifestations of dementia, such as experiencing forgetfulness or spatial recognition problems, occur in an individual person and their response to such events will be just as individual. Recognizing, identifying and ascribing such manifestations to the early signs of dementia and to a need to seek medical help is, for the person undergoing this transitional adjustment, not a straightforward and linear decision (Keady, Williams and Hughes-Roberts 2007; Keady *et al.* 2007; Pollitt, O'Connor and Anderson 1989). Within the context of an existing relationship, Keady and Gilliard (2002) identified a number of steps necessary for people with (undiagnosed) AD to take in order to reach an early diagnosis (p.22, slightly abridged):

- a self-recognition by the person with (undiagnosed) AD that 'something is wrong'
- a willingness by the person with (undiagnosed) AD openly to disclose their fears, concerns and coping behaviours
- a mutual validation of these concerns
- a decision to 'do something about it' and place the presentation within an illness (rather than an ageing) context
- primary care teams then taking the reported signs and symptoms seriously, and having the necessary knowledge and skills to facilitate an early diagnosis of AD
- the person with AD and their support network being informed about and understanding the diagnosis and prognosis.

Numerous studies have suggested that acquiring AD (or other types of dementia) at any stage of the life-cycle has a significant impact upon the person, their family and their social network (for a review see Steeman *et al.* 2006). Within this dynamic there will be individual differences in coping and adaptation due to the interaction between the person's personality style, their biography and life experiences (Clare 2002; Keady and Gilliard 1999; Woods 2001). However, at present, there appears to be limited understanding on the interrelationship and connectedness between *biography* → *coping / adaptive strategies* → *day-to-day decision-making* and it is this chain that we will now explore through the exemplar of bridging and longitudinal immersion in the post-diagnostic experience of four people with AD.

STUDY DESIGN

The primary aims of the study were twofold: first, to explore transitions through the early diagnosis of AD and further understand the person's ways of living day-by-day, including an emphasis on tracking decision-making; second, to document such change over time in the context of a constructivist grounded theory (Charmaz 2000) so that the 'mutual creation of knowledge by the viewer and viewed' (p.510) sits at the heart of the research enterprise and act. Participants were recruited through a memory clinic in North Wales where JH-R (co-author) practises as a specialist nurse, both unit and community-based. All research interviews were conducted by JH-R with data collection integrated into routine monthly home visits following the principles of practitioner research (Reed and Procter 1995). Accordingly, the study was longitudinal in design and adopted some elements of life-story work to inform the data collection process using the framework developed by Gubrium (1993).

The study was conducted with four people with an early diagnosis of AD (age range 57–78 years) over a period of 18–20 months (although JH-R's clinical contact with each of the participants continued for much longer). Data generation consisted of 80 practitioner-research contacts, 71 of those facilitating documented research contact. A method of process consent was adopted at each clinical/research contact to ensure willingness to participate and understanding of the aims of the project (Dewing 2002). All necessary ethical and research governance considerations were provided for the study and participants' names have been changed to protect anonymity.

About the participants

As this study and analysis of decision-making is built from the experience of four people living through the onset of AD, a brief outline of each of the participants is set out below:

Sarah is a 70-year-old woman who was an only child and 'brought up in the old-fashioned way, when children were seen and not heard'. She was widowed after an unhappy marriage. Sarah was diagnosed with AD in September 2002 and currently lives on her own. She cared for her father who had 'senile dementia'.

June is a 66-year-old woman who lives with her husband James. She was diagnosed with AD in January 2003. June and her husband James have a very strong, loving and close relationship and have been together for almost 50 years, as they explained: 'Our marriage is a partnership, we do everything together, we cope together.' June's philosophy of life is to take things 'one day at a time'. June has a family history of younger onset AD.

Carys is a 57-year-old woman who lives with her husband Tom; they have no children. Carys was diagnosed with AD in May 2002 and describes one of the happiest moments in her life as 'when I got married'. She worked in a bank most of her life until she encountered difficulties in counting money and constructed this early encounter with AD as 'making mistakes'. Her approach to life is to 'change what you can, be as happy as you can and if you can't change things don't worry about them'.

Peter is a 78-year-old man who lives with his wife Susan; they have two children. Peter served in the air force during his working life. He now enjoys his retirement and approaches daily life by 'just getting on with it' and feels that the way they manage every day is 'helped by our past experiences'. Peter was diagnosed with AD in April 2003.

'BRIDGING': FACILITATING DECISION-MAKING IN AD

By constantly comparing and analysing the four longitudinal life-story narratives, a number of unifying and transcending storylines emerged. Specifically, the early journey through AD was seen by each participant as consisting of three temporal stages, namely Losing Balance→Finding Balance→Keeping Balance, with decisions continually taken during each stage and at the time of a transition from one stage to the next – a process we have named 'bridging'. We will further embellish each of these three stages with reference to the story of each participant.

1. Losing Balance

This refers to the pre-diagnostic stage of AD where the (undiagnosed) signs have emerged but are integrated (with increasing difficulty) into the life-story of each individual, and their family/collective biography. Participants described this initial, and subsequently enduring, collection of signs as including:

- difficulty in calculating money and adding up
- forgetting names
- word-finding problems
- feeling apprehensive for no good reason

- olfactory changes
- losing keys and other personal items
- doing 'silly things', for example being unable to locate the car after parking in a supermarket car park
- problems mastering new technology, such as a mobile phone or a DVD player.

Each of the four participants in this study independently constructed the challenges posed by these early signs as 'making mistakes'. The following descriptions from June and Carys best summarize this initial period of uncertainty and the biographical disruption it caused.

My earliest awareness of the condition started with me feeling terrible, I didn't like my husband going out without me. I blew up. I was ashamed of my behaviour. I could have hurt him. I was never like that. I loved my children and grandchildren – they used to ask me to babysit – I just couldn't do it any more. I was really nasty with them. I felt trapped in the house. You feel it building up in your stomach. Your mouth goes dry. It's an awful feeling, you feel like exploding. (June)

When the illness first started I didn't realize anything was wrong; it was the people around me who noticed. I knew I wasn't working as well as I should be. I started making mistakes, I wasn't remembering up-to-date stuff, I remember we had a bank charge for invoicing which was always £6 and it went up to £7 and I just couldn't remember the change to £7 and that was the kind of thing that was jumped upon. Everything I did was wrong, I felt stupid and I retreated into my shell. I felt everybody was talking about me; people were out to get me. It made me feel terrible. I felt my life was being pulled apart. My husband and I thought it might be because of 'the change' at first. There were other signs as well, it wasn't just my memory, it was more than my memory, and it affected my senses. I remember one day sitting in my front room and smelling fish and chips! The worst of all it was affecting my relationship with my husband; I was increasingly taking my worries out on him. (Carys)

As can be seen from the two illustrations, prior to diagnosis the meaning of events that constitute 'making mistakes' can result in the decision to 'blame others' and 'hit out' at those who love you the most; a human failing perhaps, but one that can cause recrimination and heighten stress within family relationships. In many ways, these initial signs can involve a dissonance and separation between past and present life, an effect that intensifies with the passing of chronological time. Accordingly, decision-making can be fractured and self-centred with the person with (undiagnosed) AD looking to preserve identity and selfhood. It is only when the symptoms are placed within an illness context (i.e. what's wrong with me?) that decisions can be taken to seek an explanation and enter a stage of Finding Balance in life.

2. Finding Balance

This stage constitutes a sense of needing to know 'what's wrong with me?' without necessarily acknowledging 'what it could be'. Finding Balance requires a decision by the person with (undiagnosed) AD and/or others (partners/close family) to 'push' the issue into the open based upon recognition of difficulties and a life in crisis. All four participants spoke of the importance of receiving a diagnosis of AD and the fact that this helped (eventually in Peter's case) to recover a sense of balance and equilibrium in their life:

> When I was diagnosed [with AD] it was important to me that I was told. I had an idea anyway, because my father had dementia. I've had tremendous support from Chris and my sons so I'm not alone. (Sarah)

> Seeing the right people and finding out what was wrong. That's all we wanted. (June)

> Initially, my GP was reluctant to refer me to the memory clinic. He told us: 'You know when you have AD, it's when you can't cook the evening meal.' We had two visits there and then we were referred to the memory clinic. The doctor there did a few more tests and then we got the diagnosis. We knew where we were then; it's a pity it didn't happen earlier. (Carys)

> I have found it very difficult coming to terms with the diagnosis; I didn't want to believe it at first. At first we decided to tell only close family members and the diagnosis was not general knowledge. Gradually, we decided to tell more people. Over the past three years my memory has become worse. I've got insight into my situation and it's not much fun. However, I am still relieved I can do most things. I know I have to make allowances for my limitations. If we were to go to a lot of new places now it would be confusing, but I would still go on holiday with my daughter and son-in-law if they asked. We try and keep active. We think that's impor-tant, exercise and routine in particular. (Peter)

A recurring theme in the life-stories was the experience of receiving a diagnosis. The usual and accepted practice in memory clinics of undertaking a neurological assessment was not always seen in a positive light by those on its receiving end. For example, Sarah felt that the meaning and purpose of certain assessment tools were not always fully explained to her, and in a language she could understand; so there was little opportunity to make a decision over whether or not to go ahead with performing the test. As Sarah neatly put it, 'You had to do what you were asked.' Participants in this study wanted the choice to have their neuropsychological assessments conducted at home where they could exert some influence over the direction, timing and sharing of the procedures.

Over and above such concerns, however, the diagnosis of AD led to a new and intense experience of 'bridging' where past events were reconstructed, the present re-engineered for additional support and future decision-making approached through a new-found confidence and self-assurance. As Sarah stated, 'I'm glad that you people did give the diagnosis, because I'm coping, I'm not worrying about it.'

The diagnosis prepares the ground for entering the third stage in the model, Keeping Balance.

3. Keeping Balance

In this stage, AD and ongoing decision-making is set within the context of a life journey where events are to be lived with or fought against, key relationships valued/re-valued, and a sense of togetherness affirmed/reaffirmed. A diagnosis of AD may not be the most significant part of a life course and Sarah, for one, firmly believed that surviving her abusive marriage was by far the most defining part of her life-story. Indeed, Sarah approached her AD through feelings of self-growth and discovery:

> Although I live alone I'm not alone. And I just love my life at the moment. I go to the day centre and I love it there. And I get on well with the older people there. Because I like older people, I always have done, they fascinate me. I know the illness will progress so I do everything now; I live life to the full. I try not to look too far ahead. I tell people I have Alzheimer's disease. It's nothing to be ashamed of and we all know where we stand. I tend to make a joke of it or it would get to me. I understand that if I make mistakes it's normal. Other people will need to accept me for what I am. I can still do things, even new things.

As the title of this third stage intimates, Keeping Balance has movement and momentum, a process best captured by Carys as follows: 'One minute you are up and feeling good, the next you are down and wondering what it's all about.'

Keeping Balance involves active decision-making by the person with AD to continually test and re-test their value/coping system, as the following final summaries attest.

> **Sarah**: Her current life, five years after the diagnosis, is one of acceptance, understanding and living with her memory in a positive manner. She is facing her AD on her own, but does receive important support from services, such as the local day centre, memory clinic or visits from JH-R. There is little doubt that confirmation of the diagnosis has helped Sarah to associate the changes she is experiencing with a 'named condition'. Sarah is now able to understand and accept the changes she has been experiencing and whilst she continues to 'make mistakes', she now accepts 'it's the way I am now' and can appreciate that 'it's not my fault'. As a result she has learnt to live and cope with her life and make decisions that continue to bridge and fulfil her quality of life.
>
> **June**: After the diagnosis June and James made the decision to be open about June's AD, both at a personal level and in sharing the diagnosis with other people. As June stated: 'I'm still my normal self, I can still do things, I'm still a person.' June and James are now able to associate the emotional changes and forgetfulness with the AD. Decision-making is taken in the 'here and now' without trying to delve too much into the future, as June indicates: 'I'm not trying to avoid the issue, but I just live for today and be happy, there's no point worrying about the future.' Decision-making is performed by June and James to enable them both to maintain a sense of control over their life, a philosophy that is driven by accepting that changes have occurred and making the decision to live as normal life as possible. As June stated in her straightforward way: 'I'm not going to hide away.'
>
> **Carys**: After the diagnosis, Carys felt her life was 'back together again' and summarized her approach to life and decision-making with these words:
>
> > After the diagnosis our relationship improved and it's okay again because we now know what was causing the changes that were happening to me. We have developed a number of ways to help me cope with my poor memory; we use a blackboard and yellow stickers, which you need to

> move every couple of weeks because I stop seeing them! Keeping active is important and we go on plenty of holidays if we can. We have started telling people as well. I think that helps. We take each day as it comes. There are good and bad days, we call them 'blips'. We've noticed a few more little changes just recently, nothing really to worry about, a pointer for the future. The day club has been a great help. We are able to share things with other people who are going through the same problems. As regards the medication, we were told it would keep me on an even keel for a period of time, but I do feel better since I've started taking them; my memory is sharper, my concentration is better.

Carys and Tom are very much partners in the process of living with AD, and decision-making is seen as a joint responsibility propelled by a lifetime of togetherness and mutual love and respect for one another.

Peter: Peter's life is now about living positively with dementia. He has regained a degree of control in his life by accepting his diagnosis and making allowances for his limitations. He feels his past life experiences have been important in helping him cope in a positive manner. The support of his wife and family has also been significant in helping Peter to come to terms with his illness, as he explains:

> I still enjoy my life, I'm quite happy. We are well supported, we have a good marriage, and we are a partnership! The way we handle ourselves now is helped by our past experiences. I have a past background that has helped to prepare me for now. It was also the way we were brought up so we just 'get on with it'.

Peter and his wife remain active in the community and, as can be seen from Peter's words, day-to-day life and decision-making are shaped by his biography and philosophy of life. It is a combination of these two value bases, coupled to close family support, which enables bridging to occur and successfully help Peter on his journey.

DISCUSSION

In our opinion, the development of 'bridging' viewed through the lens of Losing Balance→Finding Balance→Keeping Balance provides an accessible theoretical account of the complexities of adjustment and decision-making in AD. Moreover, as a constructivist grounded theory (Charmaz 2000), the model identifies bridging as an ever-present process (i.e. as part of journeying through AD and rooted in biography and relationship sets). Bridging is therefore dynamic and, as the metaphor suggests, is subject to support or collapse dependent upon a range of situational and contextual conditions. We have called these conditions 'strong' and 'weak' bridging.

Strong bridging suggests a positive process by engagement in decision-making and/or actions at all points in time in the journey through AD. Of particular importance is the nature of constructed self-identity linked to biography, the account of one's life history and the strength of key relationships, such as the case of Sarah and her identity of being a 'survivor' through an abusive marriage. In such instances, decision-making through AD is primarily associated with a well-developed sense of self and personal identity, with AD contributing towards a well-rounded quality of life. In many respects this type of biographical information is central to the success of bridging; indeed, it could be described as being both biography-centred and relationship-centred. The conditions necessary for 'strong' bridging to occur could also be couched in terms of psychological and social support, as it involves being able to: access close, meaningful relationships; develop friendships with others (such as staff at the memory clinic or the day club); expect others to retain an interest in the personhood of the individual and their life history; and foster a sense of identity negotiated and reinforced through loving and close relationships.

Weak bridging denotes frailties in the lived journey through dementia due to difficulties with actions and/or failure to engage in supportive decision-making, such as accessing relevant assistance or advice at critical points in time. This failure may be due to a range of situational or conditional factors, for instance the re-treading of previous biographical 'footprints' of poor adaptation/coping/relationships, and/or being unable to access reliable or trusted sources of information. The disruption at the onset of AD and the mismatch of meaning attributed to the (undiagnosed) early signs is an example of weak bridging within the family unit. This was exemplified by Peter's initial difficulty in assimilating the diagnosis of AD into his life-story and June being 'nasty' to loved family members. This weak bridging required external support/decision-making to help 'prop up' the (undiagnosed) person's sense of identity whilst recognizing and responding to individual–family adjustment difficulties.

Locating the meaning of bridging and decision-making requires embracing discourse, empathy and narrative-based types of support and understanding. More importantly, shifting the dialogic of the personal pronoun 'I' to one of 'We', that is 'We are living with AD' (even for people who live alone with the condition, such as Sarah), is an important step in providing strong bridging for people living with AD and their families/support network. Minimizing the biographical and chronological time that people with (undiagnosed and then diagnosed) AD spend in the stages of Losing Balance and Finding Balance, whilst maximizing their time in the stage of Keeping Balance, are, we would suggest, service, policy and personal goals that should help define negotiated, meaningful and shared decision-making in the journey through AD.

ACKNOWLEDGEMENTS

This research was funded by a grant from the North Wales Research Committee. We thank the participants in the study who shared their lives, time and experiences with us all.

REFERENCES

Banerjee, S. and Chan, J. (2008) 'Organization of old age psychiatric services.' *Psychiatry, 7,* 2, 49–54.

Care Services Improvement Partnership (2005) *Everybody's Business: Integrated Mental Health Services for Older Adults: A Service Development Guide.* London: Care Services Improvement Partnership.

Charmaz, K. (2000) 'Grounded Theory: Objectivist and Constructivist Methods.' In N.K. Denzin and Y.S. Lincoln (eds) *Handbook of Qualitative Research* (2nd edn). Thousand Oaks, CA: Sage.

Clare, L. (2002) 'Developing awareness about awareness in early-stage dementia: The role of psychosocial factors.' *Dementia 1,* 3, 295–312.

Department of Health (2001) *National Service Framework for Older People: Modern Standards and Service Models.* London: HMSO.

Department of Health (2008) *Transforming the Quality of Dementia Care: Consultation on a National Dementia Strategy.* London: HMSO.

Dewing, J. (2002) 'From ritual to relationship: A person-centred approach to consent in qualitative research with older people who have dementia.' *Dementia 1,* 2, 157–171.

Gubrium, J.R. (1993) *Speaking of Life: Horizons of Meaning for Nursing Home Residents.* Newbury Park, CA: Sage.

Keady, J. and Gilliard, J. (1999) 'The Early Experience of Alzheimer's Disease: Implications for Partnership and Practice.' In T. Adams and C. Clarke (eds) *Dementia Care: Developing Partnerships in Practice.* London: Baillière Tindall.

Keady, J. and Gilliard, J. (2002) 'Testing Times: The Experience of Neuropsychological Assessment for People with Suspected Alzheimer's Disease.' In P.B. Harris (ed.) *The Person with Alzheimer's Disease: Pathways to Understanding the Experience.* Baltimore, MD: Johns Hopkins University Press.

Keady, J., Williams, S. and Hughes-Roberts, J. (2007) '"Making mistakes": Using co-constructed inquiry to illuminate meaning and relationships in the early adjustment to Alzheimer's disease – A single case study approach.' *Dementia 6,* 3, 343–364.

Keady, J., Williams, S., Hughes-Roberts, J., Quinn, P. and Quinn, M. (2007) '"A Changing Life": Co-Constructing a Personal Theory of Awareness and Adjustment to the Onset of Alzheimer's Disease.' In M. Nolan, E. Hanson, G. Grant and J. Keady (eds) *User Participation Research in Health and Social Care: Voices, Values and Evaluation.* Maidenhead: Open University Press/McGraw-Hill.

National Institute for Health and Clinical Excellence/Social Care Institute for Excellence (2006) *Dementia: Supporting People with Dementia and their Carers in Health and Social Care.* NICE Clinical Practice Guideline 42. London: National Institute for Health and Clinical Excellence.

Pollitt, P.A., O'Connor, D.W. and Anderson, I. (1989) 'Mild dementia: Perceptions and problems.' *Ageing and Society 9,* 261–275.

Pratt, R. and Wilkinson, C. (2001) *'Tell Me the Truth': Views from People with Dementia on the Impact of Being Told the Diagnosis of Dementia.* London: Mental Health Foundation.

Reed, J. and Procter, S. (1995) *Practitioner Research in Health Care: The Inside Story.* London: Chapman and Hall.

Steeman, E., Dierckx de Casterlé, B., Godderis, J. and Grypdonck, M. (2006) 'Living with early-stage dementia: A review of qualitative studies.' *Journal of Advanced Nursing 54,* 6, 722–738.

Woods, R.T. (2001) 'Discovering the person with Alzheimer's disease: Cognitive, emotional and behavioural aspects.' *Aging and Mental Health 5,* Supplement 1, S7–S16.

CHAPTER 12

Personhood, Dementia and the Use of Formal Support Services

Exploring the Decision-Making Process

DEBORAH O'CONNOR AND ELIZABETH KELSON

Supporting persons with dementia and their family carers is a high priority. Formal community support services have been developed both to help maximize the functional autonomy and quality of life of persons with dementia, and to help reduce the strain of family caregiving. These supports may include home-making services, in-home or outside-the-home respite, personal care services, day programs and caregiver support groups. Although by no means conclusive, research suggests that supportive interventions have the potential to improve the family's ability to provide care, decrease the health and mental health risks associated with caring, and delay institutionalization of the person with dementia (see for example Mittelman 2005; Schulz *et al.* 2002; Sorensen, Pinquart and Duberstein 2002). Achieving this potential however is a challenge. With few exceptions, research also suggests that community support services are often underutilized and/or used ineffectively by those with dementia and their families (Kadushin 2004). In order for support services to be most effective, they must be accessed earlier in the dementia experience (Gaugler *et al.* 2005) but how to promote this more timely connection remains a challenge (Carpentier and Ducharme 2005; Gaugler *et al.* 2005; Lyons and Zarit 1999).

There is poor understanding of why and how families access support services (O'Connor 1995, 1999). This can be attributed to at least three gaps in knowledge. First, much research has focused on the use of services by either the family member or the older person rather than examining how the two care partners may work together to make a decision. Second, the body of research that does examine the decision to use community support services rarely includes the perspective of persons with dementia, despite research that suggests that these individuals definitely can make meaningful contributions to decision-making (see for example work by Clare 2003; Clare *et al.* 2008; Phinney and Chesla 2003; Woods and Pratt 2005) and that their perspectives may differ from their family members' perspectives (see for example Bamford and Bruce 2000). Finally, understanding of the decision to use services has often employed a narrow, decontextualized lens that fails to capture how structural factors, such as the characteristics of the healthcare delivery system and policy and program guidelines, may facilitate or impede the decision to use support services. Summed together, the result is that research to date has often failed to capture the complexity associated with the decision-making process around the use of support services.

This chapter begins to tease out the dynamic and complex nature of the decision-making process in relation to the use of community support services. It will do this by developing a case study, drawn from a larger study that employed multiple case-study methodology to explore the interface between the personal and familial experience of dementia and the use of formal support services.[1] Data generation and analysis in this larger study is grounded by three assumptions:

1. The perceptions and experiences of persons with dementia must be included for a more comprehensive, complex understanding of the decision-making process around the use of support services.

2. Decision-making is a dynamic process taking place within a relational context.

3. Personal experiences around decision-making are shaped, at least in part, by broader organizational and societal practices and policies.

The husband and wife couple that is highlighted in this case study was interviewed both separately and together several times over a period of approximately one year. Interviews were transcribed verbatim and the transcripts were then analysed using a line-by-line categorizing strategy. All data pertaining to their decision-making process was then examined using the following questions: Who makes the decision to use support services? How is the person with dementia involved in the decision to use support services? How do issues related to cognitive capacity influence the process? How does this family negotiate difference?

The intent of this chapter will be to draw on this couple's 'story' to demonstrate the complexity of the decision to use community support services and to recognize the importance of understanding this decision as a dynamic, interactional process.

INTRODUCING MR AND MRS SMITH

Trudy and John Smith are an older couple who have been married for over 50 years. John is a retired minister and Trudy is a nurse. They live together in their self-owned bungalow in a semi-rural community; they have lived there for nearly 20 years and the house is filled with mementoes, personal items and family photographs. Prior to moving into this area, they were stationed in a variety of remote communities where John fished and ministered, and Trudy nursed and raised their children. Their marriage has been punctuated by a sense of working co-operatively together as leaders in these small communities.

They have 11 children, all of whom are a great source of pride to them. They describe family as extremely important to them, but it is also imperative to them that they are not perceived as a burden to their children. Hence, although their youngest daughter – in her mid-twenties – still lives at home and several of their children live within half an hour of the couple, John has been the primary carer since Trudy, now 70 years old, was diagnosed five years ago with Alzheimer disease (AD). When we met this couple, Trudy was in the middle stage of dementia; by the end of our involvement her dementia had worsened to the point where she required 24-hour care at home.

Looking back John believes that there were signs of his wife's memory loss at least 15 years earlier when Trudy retired from nursing when only 55 years old, because she had 'lost her confidence' in her ability to administer medications. She was subsequently diagnosed with depression, a diagnosis that never rang true with her family, and it was nearly ten years before the diagnosis of AD was made. Since her diagnosis, Trudy has been taking the anti-cholinesterase medication Aricept; with only moderate success, according to her husband. This medication is not publicly funded where they live and is quite expensive, but despite the financial strain associated with taking it and its questionable value, John is reluctant to discontinue it on the off-chance that it may be helping his wife's condition.

John has his own acute health concerns: uncontrolled diabetes has led to decreased kidney function and vision problems. Because of his failing eyesight, his ability to drive has been questioned by his physician; this is a serious threat to this couple's independence since they live in a semi-rural community a long way from amenities.

John retired from his position as a minister several years ago, and more recently he has withdrawn from his various volunteer roles in the community as a result of the demands on his time related to Trudy's dementia. John describes their living situation as very stressful: he has been overseeing the shopping and meal preparation for some time, and, increasingly, his wife relies on him for help dressing and bathing. The house is beginning to show signs of neglect and, at times, Trudy is resistant to his care efforts. John states that he can lose patience with his wife, a fact that causes him further distress. The couple attempt to capture their situation in the following interchange:

John: Well, I have my stressful moments.

Trudy: [wryly] It's mostly his wife's fault.

John: Well, no, I wouldn't say that honey, it's just –

Trudy: Well, I just don't like being, what would you say [fades off]... I just don't like other people doing my work [softly].

Despite the many challenges, John maintains that, overall, they 'muddle' through. Conveying his day-to-day philosophy of acceptance, he notes: 'Well, you know, we have to change our life according to the way things are, you know, and Trudy and I, of course, we had our dreams about how we'd spend our senior years and a lot of those things...we just have to put aside.'

This couple was referred for formal support before we met them. Although they were willing to consider the suggested services, it took well over a year before they finally agreed to implement any level of external help. This chapter will explore their decision-making process during this period. Their story will be organized around three main issues that emerged through their narratives: *Whose decision? Whose needs? Which needs?*

WHOSE DECISION?

People have been very gracious telling me what's available and offering, you know, various things. But it's not just as easy as one might think, you know... Someone to do housework? There's times when I thought it would be really helpful, but uh, it's not as simple as that, you know... It's easy to say that I should do that but it's not really quite as simple as that. (John)

From the outset, John and Trudy made it clear that the decision to use services was far more complex than one might initially anticipate. This couple was not alone in making this explicit – this message was conveyed by almost all of the participants in the larger study. In all cases, at least part of the complexity revolved around competing perspectives between the person with dementia and the family carer.

Much of the research and practical literature has examined the use of support services as though it were a decision made solely by the family carer. A theme that emerged both with this couple and in the larger study was how important the input from the person with dementia into the decision to use services was regarded by the carer. John recognizes this when he notes: 'Well, we've looked into that [services] and...Trudy does not want to have anybody come in.' Hence, services were not implemented.

With few exceptions, the person with dementia was often intensely involved and influential in the decision to use services. This was irrespective of his or her ability to fully understand the situation or the issues related to the use of services. Thus when Trudy states 'Well, I just don't, I just don't feel like I need to be looked after', John does not push the issue. Rather than considering whether she is in fact capable of making this decision, he attributes Trudy's opposition to her personal disposition, or personhood, and not to her dementia. For example, he explains that 'my wife's whole nature, her whole make-up, is to help people'. Trudy concurs with this statement, contending that housework is her domain and that she neither wants, nor sees the need for, someone else to do 'her' work. She views the use of in-home support services as an unnecessary 'invasion of privacy' which she is very clear that she doesn't want.

For over a year, Trudy's perspective resulted in an impasse. While John recognized the struggle to keep the house even minimally clean, to have somebody else come and assist would be 'objectionable to her [Trudy]'. Though he would prefer some in-home support, he is not prepared to distress his wife. Similarly, Trudy is instrumental in the decision not to use the local Adult Day Centre (ADC). Trudy tried the centre and then refused to return, because 'I like to be at home and I've got things to do at home'. John refused to push the issue, again, despite the acknowledged benefit he felt he derived from having some respite.

John summarizes the situation:

> Most days I can handle things fairly well. There are times when things sort of come to a bit of a pressure point and I really feel that I could do with some help. But mostly I think I…first of all, I love my wife dearly. You know, she's important to me. And she's been a good wife, excellent mother, wonderful companion. We've done a lot of things together…

The first point that this couple's story highlights, then, is the pivotal role that the person with dementia plays in the decision-making process. In this case, this involvement occurred irrespective of Trudy's ability fully to understand her care needs and the issues related to the use of services. In other words, it was issues pertaining to personhood, and not cognitive capacity, that were most powerful in this couple's decision-making process, at least at the outset.

WHOSE NEEDS? 'BUT UMM, I HAVE SERIOUS HEALTH ISSUES TOO…'

A second issue that dominated John and Trudy's story helps to further conceptualize the complexity associated with the decision to utilize supports: specifically, whose needs are to be addressed by the service? Arguably, an implicit assumption underpinning the decision to use community support is that this decision is made based on the needs of the person with dementia. This couple's story, like others in the larger study, clearly challenged the simplicity of this understanding. Rather, what became quite apparent was that the family carer and the person with dementia often had diverse, and sometimes competing, needs related to support.

Community support programs are designed to respond to a variety of needs. In this study, these included: respite, safety, independence, assistance with personal and daily care, socialization and activity, rehabilitation and carers' health issues. Unsurprisingly, a service could respond simultaneously to more than one identified need. For example, attendance in a day program could address the socialization needs of the person with dementia as well as provide respite to the family carer. However, in responding to one person's need, the same service could inadvertently worsen the situation for the other person. Taking the example of attending a day program a step further, in Trudy's situation, in addition to responding to her needs for stimulation and socialization, and giving John a much-needed break, this service also challenged her understanding of herself. Trudy's perception of this service was that it positioned her as someone who needed help, to be 'baby-sat', rather than maintaining her in her lifelong position as someone who helped others. She refused to attend the day program.

John and Trudy's story demonstrates the lack of clarity that can be associated with framing need and acknowledging who the actual 'client' is. Although positioned as the family carer, John himself had serious health difficulties related to uncontrolled diabetes and a heart condition. In fact, of the two, John's health was far more precarious; when we initially met him, his physician was suggesting that thrice-weekly dialysis was imminent and a referral to the health department had been initiated identifying him as the client who required assistance with home support. John did not acknowledge the support as being for him, but rather continued explicitly to frame it as an attempt to get someone to look after Trudy. Trudy, in turn, resisted this interpretation.

Interestingly – and consistent with the larger study – their story further suggests that the needs of the person with dementia, at least initially, may supersede those of the family member and that this hierarchy may be implicitly supported by others in the family. An overnight respite program was presented to this couple as a means to potentially meet both of their needs – Trudy's need for socialization and activity, and John's need for relief. Despite its availability, this service was turned down as both John and the family tried to make sense of Trudy's needs. Specifically, John worried that Trudy became upset and agitated when they were apart (a point that was disputed by Trudy) so he felt he could not use this support because 'Yeah. And it's very important for – I think, I need to respect that because she's… She needs to know where I'm at and so that hasn't worked.' When John finally reached a crisis point and decided that he might need to override his wife's desires and began the process of having Trudy admitted into respite care, the couple's eldest son stepped in and, according to John, declared, 'No. Don't do that!' The other children also responded 'You can't do that to Mom.' John then cancelled the respite arrangements. Thus, despite the fact that John was suffering from acute health problems and had been advised by multiple medical professionals to get some help caring for his wife, Trudy and the couple's children effectively blocked his attempts to access respite care. For the children, the notion of their mother in care was just too unsettling and they wanted her to remain at home.

This excerpt highlights two points. First, there is a clear prioritizing of needs within this family that results in the person with dementia being accorded higher priority, at least initially. In this situation and in others within the larger study, this changed only when the physical (note, not emotional or social) health of the primary family carer deteriorated to the point that it became life-threatening. Second, although it appears on the surface that one family member, the primary carer, is making the decision, on closer inspection the importance of input by other family members becomes more evident. Thus, at this point in the lives of this family, the inability to meet the diverse needs of John, Trudy and their children (which might also be competing and divergent) impedes the use of supports.

WHICH NEEDS? 'I JUST FEEL LIKE I'M IN THE WAY MOST OF THE TIME'

At some point in the process, the balance shifted between the care-partners in terms of the decision-making process. This was not necessarily at the point where questions or concerns regarding the decision-making capacity of the person with dementia surfaced. Typically, as in John's situation, this occurs when the health of the family carer had been sufficiently compromised. It was at that point that the family carer appeared to begin to recognize that he or she might be required to supplant the stated wishes of the family member with dementia. Often this was justified as the family carer recognized that the care of the person with dementia was dependent upon him or her remaining well enough to manage.

However, even when some of the issues related to *whose* needs would be met, tension remained regarding *which* needs to address. In particular, responding to physical/safety needs and personhood needs often emerged as opposing forces. On the one side, the language of physical and safety needs is most frequently used to frame the provision of service. For example, in the area where Trudy and John live, home care services are framed as: personal care such as bathing; medication assistance and reminders; end-of-life care; support and respite for caregivers; and monitoring and reporting of your health. Unsurprisingly, the assessment for these supports is identified as considering: health history and current health issues; ability to cope with your healthcare issues; permission to contact your family, your doctor and others involved in provision of care; medications being taken; management of daily living activities such as eating and dressing; family and social supports such as friendships, churches and other relevant groups; and income (see www.viha.ca/hcc/qa.htm). Notably missing in these descriptions are questions related to psycho-social needs. In other words, from the outset, the provision of support is framed in terms of physical and bio-medical needs. In contrast, Trudy, like many of the other people with dementia in the larger study, prioritized 'personhood' needs. For example, she notes: 'Well, I just don't feel like I need to be looked after... I'd rather be by myself than have a stranger coming in to look after me.' Later she expands upon this, noting that 'no woman likes to have somebody coming into [her home]'. Similarly, she feels that the day program has little to offer her:

> Trudy: Well I thought it was a waste of time, you know, if I had had more to do I would have been alright but –
>
> EK: Yeah. Would you be comfortable playing the piano for people?
>
> Trudy: Oh yeah.
>
> EK: Like volunteering to play the piano or something like that.
>
> Trudy: I've done that for –
>
> EK: Oh you have?
>
> Trudy: Yeah, for so many people or whatever.
>
> EK: Yeah, so that was the main thing, that there wasn't enough to do there?
>
> Trudy: Right.

While others might preface use of support in terms of more physical needs, this is not Trudy's lens. She implicitly considers the use of supports in relation to their psycho-social impact upon her.

John is left to hover, recognizing both sides. Verbalizing his dilemma he notes: 'The truth of the matter is that someone needs to be with Trudy. Trudy doesn't think that's the way it is, but I know it is. But it's important for my wife to have a sense of her own self-worth, who she is. And I consider that to be important too.' John's desire not only to keep Trudy physically safe, but also to maintain her personhood by, for example, supporting her need to feel useful, has meant that they are unable to benefit from home support services.

These instances whereby the needs of the person with dementia are prioritized in an effort to affirm their personhood, despite the potentially negative effects on the health of the carer, appear to hold until an event or incident occurs to change the situation. For John and Trudy, it was only when her increasing cognitive impairment lessened her opposition to supports that John was able to reinitiate her involvement in the Adult Day Centre. With Trudy engaged in the ADC program two days a week, John's need for some respite was met and he was able to obtain external homemaking to lessen his load.

DISCUSSION

The purpose of this chapter was to explore the decision-making process in relation to the use of formal support services when one family member has a dementia. Too frequently accessing formal supports has been examined as though it were a simple decision made by the primary carer in isolation from the person with dementia. Drawing on John and Trudy's story, however, the complexity of this decision-making process becomes more visible. Their story highlights several themes, all of which also emerged across the broader study.

First, it draws attention to the pivotal role the person with dementia plays in making this decision. This influence continues despite his or her ability fully to understand the situation or the issues related to the use of services – in other words, irrespective of the person with dementia's capability to make this decision. This finding is consistent with other emerging research that suggests the need to consider the dementia experience from a relational perspective with hidden power dynamics. For example, Dunham and Cannon (2008) draw attention to what they define as the 'paradox of power' in dementia caregiving, describing how the caregiver is simultaneously empowered and disempowered by the experience.

This 'paradox of power' was demonstrated in this case study in a number of ways. This included prioritizing Trudy's needs over John's: in this situation John's health was more volatile than Trudy's – he was essentially a ticking time-bomb while Trudy's condition was only gradually deteriorating – yet only when the situation reached an acute crisis point were John's needs afforded any level of primacy. Interestingly, it is John's perception that this interpretation of whose needs count was shared by other family members as demonstrated by their strenuous objection to the use of respite. This situation illustrates popular conceptions around dementia and health and wellness that suggest that because Trudy has dementia she cannot be considered to enjoy a superior level of health to that of her husband, despite his numerous acute and chronic medical conditions. This might be considered evidence of our hypercognitive culture, wherein nothing is more feared than dementia (Herskovits 1995; Post 2000). The result is that John works hard to minimize the impact of the dementia on Trudy, resulting in a prioritizing of her needs over his and a reluctance to take actions that might inadvertently challenge her self-image.

Taking this understanding a step further, John and Trudy's story suggests that attention to personhood can be seen as rooting this paradox. This challenges any focus on cognitive capacity as the pre-eminent factor in family decision-making. A focus on cognitive capacity assumes that the person with dementia and/or the family are able to accurately assess cognitive functioning and that this evaluation supersedes other aspects related to decision-making. This study provides some evidence to suggest that attending to issues of personhood may trump attention to considering how cognitive deterioration is impacting capacity. In other words, while 'capacity' may have important formal meanings within the legal and health professions, at the informal level attention to it may take a backseat to efforts to retain the personhood of the family member with dementia. At some level John knew that Trudy was not able to accurately understand and make decisions about the situation, but this only motivated him further to ensure that his actions protected her and that she did not feel discounted in any way.

Interestingly, this interpretation of the situation challenges the notion of personhood as an inherently positive concept vis-à-vis dementia care. Rather it reveals the textured complexity of drawing on a personhood lens for understanding the dementia experience, especially in relation to decision-making. Specifically, if personhood is defined as 'a standing or status that is bestowed upon one human being, by others, in the context of relationship and social being' (Kitwood 1997, p.8), then the notion of personhood disrupts mutuality within the relationship: the more dependent one person is upon the other to bestow or preserve his or her personhood, the more constrained the other person is in relation to addressing his or her own needs! Cognitive capacity is, on the other hand, arguably a cleaner notion; if one is deemed as cognitively incapable of making a particular decision, the subsequent actions demanded of the family member are clearer. Attention to personhood then 'messes up' the decision-making process at the relational level with widespread effects that impact the entire family, not all of which are positive.

Introducing the notion of personhood into the decision-making process around the use of formal support services highlights one further insight in relation to the reluctance of family members to utilize these services. As illustrated by John and Trudy's case, there is a disjuncture between the emphasis placed on this concept by the person with dementia and his or her family member and the priority it is accorded within the formal service systems. With the possible exception of day programs, which do mention socialization needs, there is usually little focus accorded to relationship or personhood needs in the language of support service delivery. In other words, despite language that might include words such as 'dignity' and 'respect' to preface how the 'client' should be treated, the framing of services invariably draws predominantly on health and safety needs and not personhood needs. While this may change as the dementia progresses and the family situation deteriorates, at least initially this is not the language that the family is drawn to when contemplating the need for support, especially when the person with dementia is vocalizing reluctance. Research indicates that the earlier families avail themselves of support the more effective these services can be (see for example Gaugler *et al.* 2005). The prioritization of personhood in dementia by participants in this study suggests the need to tailor support services better to address the unique needs of the person with dementia if this earlier access is to be realized. This finding parallels the formal, institutional dementia care experience whereby families and others are driving the shift away from solely a bio-medical focus toward more individualized care that affirms personhood. Increasingly, a more holistic understanding of dementia care is considered to be a marker of good care (Brooker 2004; Kitwood 1997).

Understanding the complexity associated with the decision-making process around the use of services has a number of practical implications. First, in recognizing this decision as extraordinarily complex, greater assistance must be provided to families around considering their options. In particular, families may need transitioning support to help them effectively use support – several participants in this study, John and Trudy included, noted how much they appreciated a periodic telephone check-in from a healthcare professional. Current trends to rely upon family members to initiate service use may not be sufficient. Second, more attention is required to examine how support programs can be framed and offered in a way that is individualized and person-centred, and that moves beyond a simplistic focus on the bio-medical. Finally, the importance of the person with dementia in this decision cannot be underestimated.

ENDNOTE

1.   This study was funded through the Alzheimer's Society of Canada in partnership with the Canadian Nurses Foundation, the Nursing Care Partnership of the Canadian Health Services Research Foundation, the Canadian Institute on Health Research (CIHR) Institute on Aging, and the CIHR Institute of Gender and Health (Grant # 06 108). It received ethical approval through the University of British Columbia Behavioural Ethics Board.

REFERENCES

Bamford, C. and Bruce, E. (2000) 'Defining the outcomes of community care: The perspectives of older people with dementia and their carers.' *Ageing and Society 20*, 543–570.

Brooker, D. (2004) 'What is person-centred in dementia care?' *Reviews in Clinical Gerontology 13*, 215–222.

Carpentier, N. and Ducharme, F. (2005) 'Support network transformations in the first stages of the caregiver's career.' *Qualitative Health Research 15*, 3, 289–311.

Clare, L. (2003) 'Managing threats to self: Awareness in early stage Alzheimer's disease.' *Social Science and Medicine 57*, 1017–1029.

Clare, L., Rowlands, J., Bruce, E., Surr, C. and Downs, M. (2008) '"I don't do like I used to do": A grounded theory approach to conceptualizing awareness in people with moderate to severe dementia living in long-term care.' *Social Science and Medicine 66*, 2366–2377.

Dunham, C.C. and Cannon, J.H. (2008) '"They're still in control enough to be in control": Paradox of power in dementia caregiving.' *Journal of Aging Studies 22*, 45–53.

Gaugler, J., Kane, R.L., Kane, R.A. and Newcomer, R. (2005) 'Early community-based service utilization and its effects on institutionalization in dementia caregiving.' *Gerontologist 45*, 2, 177–185.

Herskovits, E. (1995) 'Struggling over subjectivity: Debates about the "self" and Alzheimer's disease.' *Medical Anthropology Quarterly 9*, 2, 146–164.

Kadushin, G. (2004) 'Home health care utilization: A review of the research for social work.' *Health and Social Work 29*, 3, 219–244.

Kitwood, T. (1997) *Dementia Reconsidered: The Person Comes First.* Buckingham: Open University Press.

Lyons, K.L. and Zarit, S.H. (1999) 'Formal and informal support: The great divide.' *International Journal of Geriatric Psychiatry 14*, 183–196.

Mittelman, M. (2005) 'Taking care of the caregivers.' *Current Opinion in Psychiatry 18*, 6, 633–639.

O'Connor, D.L. (1995) 'Supporting spousal caregivers: Exploring the meaning of service use.' *Families in Society 76*, 5, 296–305.

O'Connor, D.L. (1999) 'Living with a memory-impaired spouse: (Re)Cognizing the experience.' *Canadian Journal on Aging 18*, 2, 211–235.

Phinney, A. and Chesla, C.A. (2003) 'The lived body in dementia.' *Journal of Aging Studies 17*, 283–299.

Post, S.G. (2000) 'The Concept of Alzheimer Disease in a Hypercognitive Society.' In P.J. Whitehouse, K. Maurer and J.F. Ballenger (eds) *Concepts of Alzheimer Disease: Biological, Clinical, and Cultural Perspectives.* Baltimore, MD: Johns Hopkins University Press.

Schulz, R., O'Brien, A., Czaja, S., Ory, M., *et al.* (2002) 'Dementia caregiver intervention research: In search of clinical significance.' *Gerontologist 42*, 5, 589–602.

Sorensen, S., Pinquart, M. and Duberstein, P. (2002) 'How effective are interventions with caregivers? An updated meta-analysis.' *Gerontologist 42*, 3, 356–372.

Woods, B. and Pratt, R. (2005) 'Awareness in dementia: Ethical and legal issues in relation to people with dementia.' *Aging and Mental Health 9*, 5, 423–429.

CHAPTER 13

Families, Dementia and Decisions

BARBARA PURVES AND JOANN PERRY

> *A family is a study in plate-tectonics, flow folding.*
> *Something inside shifts; suddenly we're closer, or apart.*
> *(Anne Michaels[1])*

A family is a network that extends within and across generations, geographic regions and time. Family patterns of interaction and decision-making reflect this richness and complexity, changing and shifting in small ways in response to the circumstances of everyday life. These patterns can be disrupted in more major ways, however, by significant positive or negative events, challenging families to find ways to re-establish equilibrium. One such event is a diagnosis of dementia.

To date, the majority of the research literature on family decision-making in the context of dementia has focused on a relatively narrow set of types of decisions including, for example, disclosure of diagnosis (Bamford *et al.* 2004; Vernooij-Dassen *et al.* 2006), transitions to different levels of care settings (Caron, Ducharme and Griffith 2006; Mead *et al.* 2005), and end-of-life care (Caron, Griffith and Arcand 2005; Forbes, Bern-Klug and Gessert 2000). Furthermore, attention is often focused on a triad comprising the person with dementia, a family member (often designated as 'family caregiver') and a healthcare professional or researcher (Hicks and Lam 1999). The complexities of interactions within such triads have themselves been the subject of research, with evidence of risk that the family caregiver's voice can be privileged, backgrounding or even silencing that of the person with dementia (Hirschman *et al.* 2005; Perry 2005), leading to calls for health practitioners and researchers alike to find ways to ensure that the voices of people with dementia are also heard in the decision-making process (Adams and Gardiner 2005; Dewing 2007).

MODELS FOR DECISION-MAKING

While this research undoubtedly goes some way in informing our understanding of issues associated with families' decisions regarding the care of their kin with dementia, Hicks and Lam (1999) have argued convincingly for the need for a model of the decision-making process regarding dementia that captures the complexities of families coping with dementia across the social course of the illness. In their review of decision-making models, they point out that most models typically assume a 'primary decision-maker or a group decision in which one authority has the final word' (p.418) and so cannot readily accommodate the kinds of decision-making processes used by families or social groups. Even Janzen's 'therapy group management' model, which encompasses a group of individuals, usually family members, who take charge of therapy for the ill person, does not fully capture the complexity of decision-making because it fails 'to define the roles of multiple actors and the nature of their relationships to each other' (Hicks and Lam 1999, p.419). Their proposed model, which was based on in-depth interviews with Chinese-American families, interviews with medical professionals and community ethnography, describes constellations of decision-makers, acknowledging the potential involvement of multiple family members, as well as the involvement of multiple professionals and service systems and taking into consideration the relationships among decision-makers. The model also recognizes variations in the nature of the decision-making process: Hicks and Lam point out that while healthcare practitioners and researchers tend to focus on the more major decisions described above, for family members the seemingly minor decisions of everyday life are also relevant to their experience of dementia and can play a part in how families approach the more major decisions. Finally, the model also includes the interaction of decision-making with larger social, cultural and economic forces.

In exploring the decision-making process in families we, like Hicks and Lam, argue that attention must be given to the way in which 'family' itself is understood and represented. That is, we see a need explicitly to identify ways of ensuring that the family as a whole is acknowledged and recognized as germane to the dialogue. Such consideration is critical in light of evidence that the repositioning of individual family members as family caregivers primarily occurs not within the family but rather through interactions with others beyond the family, including healthcare professionals, community-based support groups and researchers (O'Connor 2007). Our intent in this chapter is to explore and illustrate the complexities of family relationships in decision-making and dementia, not only within the context of healthcare decision-making, but also in the context of everyday life. In so doing, we hope to encourage others to extend this exploration in order to create a more comprehensive understanding of these issues. We begin by reviewing how the concept of family itself is represented in dementia research, followed by a discussion of methodological approaches that consider the family as a unit. We then illustrate through a single family case study how these approaches, applied to the study of a family caring for someone with dementia, can illuminate its decision-making processes in everyday life.

REPRESENTATIONS OF FAMILY IN DEMENTIA RESEARCH

The question of who or even what is family has received considerable attention in the dementia research literature over at least the past two decades (Gubrium and Holstein 1990; Keating *et al.* 1994; Montgomery and Williams 2001). While it has long been recognized that family caregiving often (if not typically) involves more than one family member (Matthews and Rosner 1988; Sims-Gould 2006; Tennstedt, McKinlay and Sullivan 1989), the relative lack of research into understanding the caregiving experience within the family as a unit has also been recognized (Dupuis and Norris 1997). Numerous studies have explored family caregiving within different types of role relationships including wives caring for husbands (Brown and Allgood 2004; Perry 2002), husbands caring for wives (Kirsi, Hervonen and Jylhä 2000, 2004; Parsons 1997; Russell 2001), daughters caring for mothers (Forbat 2003; Perry 2004; Ward-Griffin *et al.* 2007) and daughters-in-law and sons-in-law caring for their spouses' parents (Globerman 1996). Others have compared family caregiving across these different role relationships (Chesla, Martinson and Muwaswes 1994; MacRae 2002). Several studies that have included multiple family members have contributed to our understanding of tensions and negotiations within caregiving families, but their findings were discussed across families, obscuring visibility of each family as an independent unit (Garwick, Detzner and Boss 1994; Globerman 1994, 1996). While these studies have given us considerable insights into specific role relationships, understanding of the relationships within families as units remains relatively unexplored. It is our contention that research for gaining such understanding must be based on the study of particular families. Only when such a research foundation has been established will it be possible fully to explore trends across family units.

Recognition of the family as a unit invites consideration of how the family collectively makes meaning of its circumstances, necessitating understanding of how these meanings are shared (or not) among individual members. This poses methodological challenges, however, because analysis must occur at two different but related levels: that is, at the level of the individual, and at the level of the family as a social unit of interacting individuals. Perry and Olshansky (1996) addressed these challenges in a qualitative case study of a family comprising five members by drawing on Patterson's (1993) model of family meanings, which elaborated on Reiss's family paradigm of shared explanatory systems (Reiss 1981). Through in-depth interviews with all five individuals, Perry and Olshansky first identified how each one interpreted the situation of having one member with Alzheimer disease (AD). This included the following: first, the ways in which each individual saw the person with AD as being the same, or different, as he was prior to disease onset; second, identifying how, based on the meanings of what he or she saw, each individual redefined the identity of the person with AD; and, third, how each individual rewrote his or her identity with the person with AD, based on the perceived identity change. After exploring these individual meanings, Perry and Olshansky identified how differences among them precluded the family from having a shared meaning so that, ultimately, the family could not develop a unified family-coping response.

While Perry and Olshansky's study did not focus specifically on decision-making, the implications of their findings for the decision-making process in families of people with dementia is immediately clear. In addition, their study demonstrates methodologies for exploring this topic in ways that highlight the interaction between individual and family levels of meaning. The following case study further describes this process, and its impact on decision-making, in one family of a person with dementia.

CASE STUDY
Overview
Findings for this discussion of decision-making are drawn from a case study (Purves 2006) that sought to explore: first, meanings given by individual family members to their experiences of being part of a family including a person with dementia; second, how those meanings were constructed through

their talk; and third, how congruencies and contradictions among those individual meanings interacted to contribute to *family* levels of meanings, with consequences for the family as a single social unit. This focus on meanings constructed through social interaction situates the study within the theoretical framework of symbolic interactionism, described by Blumer (1969) as having three fundamental premises:

> The first premise is that human beings act toward things on the basis of the meanings they have for them... The second premise is that the meaning of such things is derived from, or arises out of, the social interaction that one has with one's fellows. The third premise is that these meanings are handled in, and modified through, an interpretative process used by the person in dealing with the things he encounters. (p.2)

Blumer's third premise, emphasizing the human capacity for reflectivity and interpretation, suggests that because individuals can conceptualize aspects of their own experience as objects of thought, meanings that these experiences hold for them can be explored through in-depth qualitative interviewing. His second premise, however, suggests the importance of additional methodologies designed to study everyday interaction itself so that we can begin to understand the process by which those meanings are created. The approaches of conversation analysis (Heritage 1984) and interactional sociolinguistics (Schiffrin 1994) provide ways for analysing talk as process.

Considerations of these different views of talk led to two methodological approaches in the present case study. The first approach, comprising in-depth interviews with each family member, provided a foundation for understanding family meanings, which at the level of the family as a social group are jointly constructed but socially distributed across individual members. The second approach comprised analysis of naturally occurring family conversations to explore how those concepts were constituted in everyday talk itself. This approach was supplemented by participant observation, which facilitated a deeper appreciation of the social context of the family.

Although decision-making was not identified as a specific topic during interviews, it emerged as a theme in several individual interviews. In addition, conversational data shed further light on how different family members approached decision-making with their kin with dementia. It is these findings that are highlighted in the following discussion.

Participants

A woman diagnosed with Alzheimer disease and her husband, identified through a local clinic, were informed about the study and invited to participate with their family. They defined this participation as including themselves and their three adult children and arranged a family meeting with the researcher after which, in accordance with ethical review board guidelines, each family member gave informed consent to participate. In the description that follows, all names are pseudonyms.

The Tanaka family included Rose and her husband Tom (both in their mid-seventies) and their three adult children, Linda, Maria and Colin (all aged between 30 and 40). The family described their mixed Japanese and Canadian heritage: both Rose and Tom were born in Canada and both spoke Japanese as well as English. However, the language of the Tanaka home was English, with the children speaking little, if any, Japanese.

All three Tanaka children lived in their own homes with their partners within a few miles of their original family home where their parents still lived. Only Colin had children: a daughter aged six years and another aged 18 months. The family was very close, describing regular visits with each other, both individually and at frequent family get-togethers. Family members supported each other in their respective businesses and in daily life. Rose had worked as a bookkeeper in several family businesses and had provided child-care for her grandchildren.

Rose's diagnosis of probable Alzheimer disease, made about six months prior to the onset of the study, was the result of a multidisciplinary assessment over the preceding several months. Results from this assessment indicated that she had a mild-moderate cognitive impairment consistent with early Alzheimer disease. Reassessment coinciding with the end of the year-long study showed progression to moderate dementia. Her family had all been aware of changes in her behaviour over one or two years that eventually led to the assessment, and all, including Rose, were aware of her diagnosis of AD.

Data collection and analysis

Individual in-depth interviews were conducted with each family member at the beginning of the study, using an open-ended question format. All interviews were recorded and transcribed for subsequent constant comparative analysis to identify patterns and themes within and across topic areas. Follow-up interviews were conducted with each family member after initial analysis and write-up of findings, first, to ensure that participants' comments were not misinterpreted and, second, to ensure that the participants were aware that other family members would be reading their comments and were willing to have those comments included. (There were no instances of family members requesting revisions or deletions.)

Conversational recordings were obtained by inviting family members to record conversations that included Rose, encouraging them to select conversations that they considered representative of their interactions together. They could choose to record conversations either with a Sony digital video-recorder or with a Sony MiniDisc player for audio-recordings. Conversational data included one video-recorded and six audio-recorded conversations, ranging in length from approximately 15 to 75 minutes. All family members participated in at least one conversation, with the number of participants ranging from two to four individuals. One conversation included the first author. Data were analysed by loading digital audio-files into the software program ATLAS.ti 5.0, with each conversation loaded as a primary document that could be segmented into quotations and subsequently coded. Analysis involved integrating the interview and conversational data: for this chapter, instances of talk in both sets of data that involve decision-making have been identified for discussion.

Findings

Transition points: Seeking a diagnosis

In the research literature on decision-making in families of people with dementia, decisions to seek or disclose a diagnosis of dementia have been identified as significant transition points in the social course of dementia. Talk about the process of diagnosis for Rose occurred only in the individual interviews (i.e. it was never a topic of recorded family conversations); nonetheless, that talk illuminated much about how the practicalities and implications of that decision affected the family as a whole.

All three adult children described how at first they individually accounted for their mother's increasing difficulty in everyday activities, such as remembering upcoming events, paying bills and adding up numbers, as expected consequences of aging and fatigue; however, as they continued to see her having problems, they collectively began to question the possibility of Alzheimer disease, albeit at different times. For example, Maria commented: 'I think my brother and my sister were a little bit more ahead than me [in articulating the possibility of Alzheimer disease].' Nevertheless, their individual reluctance to seek a diagnosis was overcome by Colin's concern for his daughter (for whom Rose was providing day-care), which he described as follows: 'I started to monitor more closely than the rest of the family, because I had my daughter to think about.' Both of Colin's sisters echoed his concerns for his daughter's safety as a prime factor in their decision to seek a diagnosis for Rose, and both described how they began to push their father to take Rose for medical assessment – an undertaking which, according to all three children, he initially resisted.

For Tom, in contrast to his children, there was not a gradual, growing awareness of something wrong, but rather a 'key thing that really got [him] going' in the form of official notification that Rose had failed to file the couple's income tax returns. Nevertheless, in his account there is even then a suggestion of resistance to interpretation of something being seriously wrong: 'You know, we do tend to forget things, it's a natural thing.' Further, he acknowledged a difference in his level of concern as compared with his children's level of caring: 'They [the kids] have been very very caring. In fact, maybe – I hate to say this – but maybe even more so than I – I tend to be a little bit…well, laid back a bit.' Although he finally agreed to take Rose for assessment, there was still not full consensus around the reasons for it. For the three adult children it was to confirm a suspicion that they did not believe their father shared, as seen in Maria's comment:

> I ended up calling and trying to get it faster, 'cause I just – I just wanted to have a label, even though you don't want a label, but you just – for my dad to know so that he wouldn't get so angry at her all the time or…you know, frustrated.

From these accounts, the pattern regarding seeking a diagnosis of dementia appeared to be one of diffuse decision-making (to draw on terminology from Hicks and Lam 1999) in which the three children united as allies in prompting Tom to act. However, a key question in this family's decision-making process concerns how they involved Rose in the discussion. No family member discussed Rose's participation in deciding whether or when to seek medical assessment. In contrast, when Rose was asked in the interview about events leading up to diagnosis, she recounted her daughters telling her: 'You're kind of…a bit…losing your memory or something.' Her response to this was relief at having her subjective impressions supported, as she recollected telling them: 'I'm glad you noticed that, because I noticed it myself.' Although it is clear from these comments that Rose was aware of her family's concern, her participation in deciding what to do about it is less clear. However, we can gain some insight into Rose's participation in decision-making by turning our attention to the smaller decisions of everyday life.

Everyday decision-making: Individual differences

Findings from both interview and conversational data bring insight into the Tanaka family's approaches to everyday decision-making with or for Rose, highlighting both similarities and differences across family members. For her husband, Tom, a significant consequence of Rose's dementia was that she no longer participated in shared decision-making about upcoming events. While he acknowledged that he rarely talked about such topics with Rose, he also explained it in terms of his approach to making decisions involving her: 'Really, there's no point in my saying what – or discussing what we should do. I've got everything planned out for her.' In his account, her lack of participation in decision-making was based on an unquestioned assumption of inability associated with her diagnosis.

Tom's assumptions about Rose's abilities to participate in decision-making were to some extent shared by other members of the family; others, however, also questioned their own part in her loss of independence. The eldest daughter, Linda, for example, commented: 'We're making all her decisions for her now, which is kind of sad.' When asked if Rose seemed to notice that, Linda described in some detail an incident in which she helped her mother to choose an outfit for a special event the next day, laying out dress, shoes and jewellery ready to be put on. The next day, her mother came to the event beautifully dressed (an attribute that Linda described her as always having had), but in a completely different outfit to the one laid out ready for her. For Linda, there was a troubling incongruence between her mother's inability to remember preparing an outfit with Linda and her unexpected ability to find 'the perfect suit, everything' – an incongruence that made her unsure of her assumptions about her mother's steadily declining capabilities.

Family conversations also revealed how Rose was involved (or not) in making decisions. During one occasion, when she was spending the afternoon with her son Colin and his daughter, the following exchange occurred:[2]

Colin: So you're going to come to swimming lessons with us.

Rose: ...Oh...is that right?

Colin: Yeah.

Rose: Last time, where – where was it that we had all that...right by that uh...little–

Colin: ...Umm #name# pool.

Rose: Yeah.

Colin: 'Cause Dad's not gonna be home, so – [conversation interrupted]

Colin's opening comment, with its final fall in intonation (indicated by a full stop), was framed, not as an invitation, but as a statement signifying a decision that had already been made. The introductory discourse marker 'so' suggests a reference to some basis for the decision, but it was not found in preceding talk – rather, it followed in Colin's explanation given in the last line of the excerpt. Rose, with her rising intonation in her first turn questioning the preceding statement, seemed to be seeking confirmation rather than challenging the decision itself (given her acceptance in her last turn).

In contrast to Tom's and Colin's tendency to make everyday decisions for Rose, both daughters made some effort to involve her in the process when they could. At a family dinner with Tom, Rose and their two daughters, Tom engaged Linda and Maria in discussion of plans for a trip to Thailand or Hawaii with Rose.

Tom: The first thing is...I've got to find out about the air, whether...uh...whether I can arrange – maybe I'll look after that.

Linda: You liked Thailand, didn't you Rose?

Tom: Yeah, I'll see if I can–

Rose: Yeah, I liked it.

Tom: So that's in the – that's in the works.

Maria (looking at Rose): Which – which one did you want to – did *you* want to – if you had a choice between Hawaii and Thailand, which one would you want to go to.

Rose (after a few seconds): Um...I like Thailand,

Maria: Mmhm...do you want to go back?

Rose: Um...because there was kind of a lot of villages, and – and things, and people were more... uh...easy to talk to,

Maria: Mmhm,

Tom: *Talk* to?

Maria (quietly): Yeah.

Linda: Well, they spoke English.

Maria: Yeah. Did you – would you prefer Thailand?...or...or...Hawaii.

Linda: Well they can do both, she can do both.

Linda, in her first turn, prompted Rose's participation by establishing both that she had been to Thailand and that she had liked it, so she might be expected to have an opinion about going there again. Rose, while acknowledging her past experience, did not take advantage of this opportunity until Maria explicitly asked about her preference, backtracking to make sure that Rose was oriented to the discussion. The following stretch of talk was characterized by a change of pace that made it stand out from the surrounding few minutes of talk. Rose's answer followed a significant pause, during which no one else spoke, nor was there any sound of background activity. Everyone present waited for Rose's response, creating a conversational space to facilitate her participation in the discussion. Yet, even given those prompts, Rose's comments about Thailand could not necessarily be taken as preference for travel there. Tom's exaggerated repetition of Rose's words ('*Talk* to?') could be interpreted as dismissive, potentially undermining Rose's credibility in knowing what she preferred. Her daughters, however, interjected with support for her comment, even though just a few minutes earlier Linda herself had suggested that Hawaii might be more relaxing because everyone spoke English and Maria had commented on additional stress in travel to Thailand associated with not knowing the language. Indeed, Rose may have been incorporating her daughters' earlier comments, albeit incorrectly, to construct a response, which possibly contributed to Tom's challenge of her ability to make an informed decision. Nonetheless, her daughters' defence of her claim, coupled with Maria's repeated question in her last turn, demonstrate a willingness to maintain at least the appearance of her participation in decision-making.

In this case study, we see that interview and conversational data both contribute to an understanding of the interaction of individual *and* family level meanings in decision-making processes. With respect to the major decision of seeking a diagnosis, retrospective interview accounts show that the individual voices of the three adult children, relatively cohesive from the outset, truly united as a single voice to convince their father of the need to seek diagnosis. Ultimately, this led to acceptance of Rose's diagnosis of dementia as a shared family meaning. The conversational data, in contrast, highlight the *process* of interaction of individual voices in the family's approach to everyday decision-making for and with Rose. In exploring this process, we see differences across family members, with Rose's husband Tom and her son Colin excluding her from the decision-making process in conversation, while her two daughters (in particular, Maria) seek to facilitate her participation, at least to the extent of inviting her opinions.

Discussion

For families, a diagnosis of dementia can represent a major shift in the 'plate-tectonics' of everyday life. Such a shift necessarily involves creating new meanings not only for each individual but also for the family as a whole because, as Blumer contends, people within a society (or, in this case, a family) must meet situations thrust on them by 'working out joint actions in which participants have to align their acts to one another' (1966, p.541). It is these joint actions in everyday life that both shape and are shaped by the interaction of individual and shared family meanings; it is the congruity of meanings informing these joint actions that determines whether families become closer or further apart.

Analysis of the Tanaka family data illustrates clearly how some meanings around decision-making can become reified, represented in interviews as 'the way it is' (e.g. Tom's assertion and acceptance of needing to plan everything for Rose, which represented the dominant family view). At the same time, there is also evidence of the ongoing processes involved in creating and modifying meanings (exemplified in Linda's description of an event that led to troubling questions of assumptions about her mother's ability). These findings highlight how the reification of family meanings, which could lead in this case to an overextension of assumptions of incapacity, can be challenged by individual voices. Analysis of family conversations provides further evidence of how differences in individual meanings that may seem fairly subtle can lead to very different styles and goals of conversational interactions. This is exemplified by Linda's and Maria's efforts to seek their mother's opinion in making decisions in contrast to Tom's and Colin's patterns of exclusion.

These findings raise further important questions regarding the participation of a person with dementia in family decision-making. Specifically, it is important to recognize that conversations inviting input from persons with dementia may give those persons voice, but they do not necessarily give them choice. For some decisions, this is perhaps as it must be: if the person's judgment is sufficiently compromised to preclude choice in some decisions, inclusion in the decision-making conversation means at least that he or she is not silenced completely. This, if combined with decision-making made by a caring family that takes the person's preferences into account whenever possible, may be as much as one can hope for.

The challenge and the dilemma for each and every family is, of course, to know which decisions are which. While we can generalize the nature of this dilemma across families, we cannot generalize the nature of the experience of any particular family. For example, findings from the Tanaka family, in which family-level meanings are interwoven with individually nuanced meanings to create a relatively cohesive family unit, stand in obvious contrast to the more fractured meaning structure of the family in Perry and Olshansky's (1996) paper. Clearly, in order to gain a more comprehensive understanding of family decision-making in caring for persons with dementia, there is a need for more research focusing on the family as a social unit. While there are substantial challenges in conducting such research, there is also great potential for identifying issues and strategies that more fully represent families' experiences and, as a result, more appropriately address their needs in the complex process of decision-making.

ENDNOTES

1. Excerpted from the poem 'Miner's Pond' in *The Weight of Oranges/Miner's Pond* by Anne Michaels (1997), published by McClelland & Stewart Ltd. Used with permission of the publisher.

2. Transcription used in analysis has been simplified here for readability. Note that the three-point dots ('…') indicate a brief pause.

REFERENCES

Adams, T. and Gardiner, P. (2005) 'Communication and interaction within dementia care triads.' *Dementia 4*, 2, 185–205.

Bamford, C., Lamont, S., Eccles, M., Robinson, L., May, C. and Bond, J. (2004) 'Disclosing a diagnosis of dementia: A systematic review.' *International Journal of Geriatric Psychology 19*, 151–169.

Blumer, H. (1966) 'Sociological implications of the thought of George Herbert Mead.' *American Journal of Sociology 71*, 535–548.

Blumer, H. (1969) *Symbolic Interactionism: Perspective and Method.* Englewood Cliffs, NJ: Prentice-Hall.

Brown, J.W. and Allgood, M.R. (2004) 'Realizing wrongness: Stories of older wife caregivers.' *Journal of Applied Gerontology 23*, 2, 104–119.

Caron, C., Ducharme, F. and Griffith, J. (2006) 'Deciding on institutionalization for a relative with dementia: The most difficult decision for caregivers.' *Canadian Journal on Aging 25*, 2, 193–205.

Caron, C., Griffith, J. and Arcand, M. (2005) 'End-of-life decision making in dementia: The perspective of family caregivers.' *Dementia 4*, 1, 113–136.

Chesla, C., Martinson, I. and Muwaswes, M. (1994) 'Continuities and discontinuities in family members' relationships with Alzheimer's patients.' *Family Relations 45*, 5–9.

Dewing, J. (2007) 'Participatory research: A method for process consent with persons who have dementia.' *Dementia 6*, 1, 11–25.

Dupuis, S. and Norris, J.E. (1997) 'A multidimensional and contextual framework for understanding diverse family members' roles in long-term care facilities.' *Journal of Aging Studies 11*, 4, 297–325.

Forbat, L. (2003) 'Relationship difficulties in dementia care.' *Dementia 2*, 1, 67–84.

Forbes, S., Bern-Klug, M. and Gessert, C. (2000) 'End-of-life decision making for nursing home residents with dementia.' *Journal of Nursing Scholarship 32*, 3, 251–258.

Garwick, A.W., Detzner, D., and Boss, P. (1994) 'Family perceptions of living with Alzheimer's disease.' *Family Process 33*, 327–340.

Globerman, J. (1994) 'Balancing tensions in families with Alzheimer's disease: The self and the family.' *Journal of Aging Studies 8*, 2, 211–232.

Globerman, J. (1996) 'Motivations to care: Daughters- and sons-in-law caring for relatives with Alzheimer's disease.' *Family Relations 45*, 37–45.

Gubrium, J.R. and Holstein, J.A. (1990) *What is Family?* Mountainview, CA: Mayfield.

Heritage, J. (1984) *Garfinkel and Ethnomethodology.* Cambridge: Polity Press.

Hicks, M.H.R. and Lam, M.S.C. (1999) 'Decision-making within the social course of dementia: Accounts by Chinese-American caregivers.' *Culture, Medicine, and Psychiatry 23*, 415–452.

Hirschman, K.B., Joyce, C.M., James, B.D., Xie, S.X. and Karlawish, J.H.T. (2005) 'Do Alzheimer's disease patients want to participate in a treatment decision, and would their caregivers let them?' *The Gerontologist 45*, 3, 381–388.

Keating, N.C., Kerr, K., Warren, S., Grace, M. and Wertenberger, D. (1994) 'Who's the family in family caregiving?' *Canadian Journal on Aging 13*, 2, 268–287.

Kirsi, T., Hervonen, A. and Jylhä, M. (2000) 'A man's gotta do what a man's gotta do: Husbands as caregivers to their demented wives: A discourse analytic approach.' *Journal of Aging Studies 14*, 2, 153–169.

Kirsi, T., Hervonen, A. and Jylhä, M. (2004) 'Always one step behind: Husbands' narratives about taking care of their demented wives.' *Health: An Interdisciplinary Journal for the Social Study of Health, Illness, and Medicine 8*, 2, 159–181.

MacRae, H. (2002) 'The identity maintenance work of family members of persons with Alzheimer's disease.' *Canadian Journal on Aging 32*, 3, 405–415.

Matthews, S.H. and Rosner, T. (1988) 'Shared filial responsibility: The family as the primary caregiver.' *Journal of Marriage and the Family 50*, 185–195.

Mead, L.C., Eckert, K., Zimmerman, S. and Schumacher, J.G. (2005) 'Sociocultural aspects of transitions from assisted living for residents with dementia.' *The Gerontologist 45* (Special Issue 1), 15–123.

Montgomery, R.J.V. and Williams, K.N. (2001) 'Implications of differential impacts of care-giving for future research on Alzheimer care.' *Aging and Mental Health 5*, Supply 1, S23–S34.

O'Connor, D. (2007) 'Self-identifying as a caregiver: Exploring the positioning process.' *Journal of Aging Studies 21*, 165–174.

Parsons, K. (1997) 'The male experience of caregiving for a family member with Alzheimer's disease.' *Qualitative Health Research 7*, 3, 391–407.

Patterson, J.M. (1993) 'The Role of Family Meanings in Adaptation to Chronic Illness and Disability.' In A.P. Turnbull, J.M. Patterson, S.K. Behr, D.L. Murphy, J.G. Marquis and

M.J. Blue-Banning (eds) *Cognitive Coping, Families, and Disability*. Baltimore, MD: Paul H. Brookes.

Perry, J. (2002) 'Wives giving care to husbands with Alzheimer's disease: A process of interpretive caring.' *Research in Nursing and Health 25*, 307–316.

Perry, J. (2004) 'Daughters giving care to mothers who have dementia: Mastering the 3 R's of (re)calling, (re)learning, and (re)adjusting.' *Journal of Family Nursing 10*, 1, 50–69.

Perry, J. (2005) 'Expanding the dialogue on dementia: (Re-)positioning diagnosis and narrative.' *Canadian Journal of Nursing Research 37*, 2, 166–180.

Perry, J. and Olshansky, E.F. (1996) 'A family's coming to terms with Alzheimer's disease.' *Western Journal of Nursing Research 18*, 1, 12–28.

Purves, B. (2006) *Family Voices: Analyses of Talk in Families with Alzheimer's Disease or a Related Disorder*. Unpublished PhD dissertation, University of British Columbia, Vancouver.

Reiss, D. (1981) *The Family's Construction of Reality*. Cambridge, MA: Harvard University Press.

Russell, R. (2001) 'In sickness and in health: A qualitative study of elderly men who care for wives with dementia.' *Journal of Aging Studies 15*, 351–367.

Schiffrin, D. (1994) *Approaches to Discourse*. Cambridge, MA: Blackwell.

Sims-Gould, J. (2006) *Family Caregiving or Caregiving Alone: Who Helps the Helper?* Unpublished PhD dissertation, University of British Columbia, Vancouver.

Tennstedt, S.L., McKinlay, J.B. and Sullivan, L.M. (1989) 'Informal care for frail elders: The role of secondary caregivers.' *The Gerontologist 29*, 5, 677–683.

Vernooij-Dassen, M., Derksen, E., Scheltens, P. and Moniz-Cook, E. (2006) 'Receiving a diagnosis of dementia.' *Dementia 5*, 3, 397–410.

Ward-Griffin, C., Oudshoorn, A., Clark, K. and Bol, N. (2007) 'Mother–adult daughter relationships within dementia care: A critical analysis.' *Journal of Family Nursing 13*, 1, 13–32.

CHAPTER 14

The Communicative Capacity of the Body and Clinical Decision-Making in Dementia Care

PIA C. KONTOS AND GARY NAGLIE

INTRODUCTION

The principles of person-centred care have been widely espoused in a range of care environments (Henderson and Vesperi 1995; Kitwood 1997; Nolan, Booth and Nolan 1997). The central premise of person-centred care is that the knowledge of a person – their preferences, capabilities and characteristics – should inform clinical decision-making (McCormack 2004; Whittemore 2000). In this sense, the core process of decision-making is using knowledge of the particulars of individual patients to make clinical judgments about strategies for their care.

Central to the care of individuals with advanced dementia is the management of behavioural disturbances, the most common of which is agitation (Cohen-Mansfield 1996). In the context of agitation management, person-centred care is premised on the understanding that agitation is not always symptomatic of dementia but can be the expression of an unmet need of the patient (Stokes 1996). In other words, the behaviour of persons with Alzheimer's disease is not always symptomatic of dementia itself, but may instead be due to a variety of reasons, such as response to physical pain or discomfort

(Douzjian, Wilson and Shultz 1998), environmental over-stimulation (Kovach *et al.* 2004; Rader *et al.* 2006), inactivity (Dobbs *et al.* 2005) and/or social isolation (Cohen-Mansfield 2001; Geda and Rummans 1999). Person-centred dementia care focuses on potential environmental and social causes of behavioural problems in dementia (Cohen-Mansfield and Mintzer 2005) and advocates non-pharmacological interventions before resorting to the use of psychotropic medication (Fossey *et al.* 2006; Moniz-Cook, Woods and Richards 2001) to suppress or eliminate challenging behaviours (Douglas, James and Ballard 2004). This involves assessing the triggers of the behaviour and its consequences, and designing an appropriately individualized intervention (Emerson 1998).

Although long-term care programs across Canada now mandate person-centred approaches to care (Chan and Kenny 2001), closer examination of practice settings discloses a very different picture. The treatment and management of behavioural problems continues to be endorsed by institutional policies of control and containment (i.e. combinations of environmental, mechanical or pharmacological restraint) (Andrews 2006). Large proportions of nursing home residents with dementia receive tranquillizers for behavioural symptoms (Bronskill *et al.* 2004; Rochon *et al.* 2007) despite evidence of only modest efficacy, high placebo response (DeDeyn *et al.* 1999; Street *et al.* 2000) and serious adverse consequences (Sink, Holden and Yaffe 2005).

Staff shortages, increasing workloads and the related insufficiency of time are commonly cited as the sources of the deficiency in quality of care (Hall and Kiesners 2005; Mark 2002). While the consequences of inadequate staffing are not to be disputed, in addition to low staffing ratios, it is our contention that a limitation of person-centred methods of care influences the quality of care provided. Person-centred approaches to care are limited in that they overlook the importance of the body, its gestures and movements, for the expression of selfhood by persons with severe cognitive impairment (Hubbard *et al.* 2002). In cases of severe cognitive impairment, the body is the fundamental means of engaging with others (Kontos 2004, 2006a; Kontos and Naglie 2007a). Thus, the significance of overlooking the importance of embodied self-expression in dementia is that day-to-day decision-making regarding care is not consistent with the particulars of the person with dementia. As a consequence, behaviours can be misread as symptomatic of dementia, leading to the overuse of tranquillizers (Douglas *et al.* 2004; Margallo-Lana *et al.* 2001) and other forms of restraint, such as bed rails (Hamers, Gulpers and Strick 2004).

We wish to explore the importance of the body as an indispensable source of knowledge that should inform clinical decision-making in dementia care. Drawing upon focus group discussions with front-line healthcare practitioners, we argue that social and cultural habits, movements and other physical cues disclose significant information about the particularity of care recipients, which brings their personhood into focus for the practitioners and facilitates greater sympathetic connection. The importance of the body for self-expression has been elaborated by Kontos (2004, 2005, 2006a) in the context of her conceptualization of selfhood in Alzheimer's disease. She argues that selfhood persists even in the presence of severe cognitive impairment since it is sustained at a pre-reflective level by the primordial as well as the socio-cultural aspects of the body. In our discussion of the body's communicative capacity and its significance for clinical decision-making, we draw upon the notion of *embodied selfhood*, specifically the importance of social habits, gestures and actions for self-expression. Embodied selfhood is a notion that explicates a source of knowledge that, as we shall argue, informs practitioners' decision-making by facilitating identification that gives them sympathetic connection with their care recipients.

FOCUS GROUP STUDY

Methods[1]

Six focus groups were conducted in three academic healthcare facilities in an urban region of Ontario, Canada. The participating facilities specialize in the care of persons with dementia and provide a range of programs and services including acute inpatient care, outpatient care, complex continuing care, long-term care and rehabilitation. Each focus group participant attended a live performance of a research-based dramatic production, entitled *Expressions of Personhood in Alzheimer's*. The production consisted of five separate vignettes each portraying bodily expressions of selfhood by severely cognitively impaired residents of an Alzheimer support unit. These expressions were observed occurrences drawn from ethnographic research on an Alzheimer support unit (Kontos 2004) in a Jewish long-term care facility. The following is one of the vignettes (Kontos 2006a):

> On the eighth day of Hanukkah, a party is organized for the residents of the Alzheimer support unit. Following the celebratory lighting of the Menorah (a ceremonial candelabrum), the staff begin to return the residents to the unit when a female resident resists. She clutches the personal support worker's arm and shakes her head vehemently indicating that she does not want to go. The personal support worker is temporarily distracted by another resident. The woman struggles to make a

path for herself through the crowd, manually pushing her wheelchair to the table where the Menorah stands in glorious full flame. She carefully unfolds a napkin on which she had earlier been served a jelly donut, and places it with utmost care atop her head to cover her hair as is required at the time of prayer under Jewish law. As is typically done when lighting candles upon the beginning of the Jewish Sabbath (Shabbat), she then holds her palms up to the Menorah, embracing the warmth of the candles, and after making three sweeping motions with her hands she covers her eyes with her hands and she privately prays to herself as tears stream through her fingers. She removes the napkin that covered her head and, when staff return for her, she does not resist. Her hands are gently clasped in her lap and her face is peaceful as she leaves the room.

The vignettes were chosen for their vivid depiction of how selfhood is manifested in bodily movements and gesture (Kontos and Naglie 2006) and served as a springboard for discussion about the relevance and importance of embodied self-expression for dementia care.

The focus group discussions were based on a series of semi-structured questions about participants' reactions to the production, specifically their understanding of self-expressions by persons with severe cognitive impairment through bodily habits and gestures, and their interpretation of the interactions between practitioners and their care recipients depicted in the staged vignettes. Participants were invited to compare and contrast what was portrayed in the production with their own experiences in order to explore self-expression by persons with severe Alzheimer's in the context of their practice, and the implications of recognizing or not recognizing such expressions for dementia care.

Participants

A purposive sampling strategy (Denzin 2000) was used to select the participants involving the following criteria for participant eligibility:

- a nurse, personal support worker, occupational therapist, physiotherapist or recreational therapist
- with experience in providing direct care (e.g. bathing, dressing, feeding, rehabilitation) to patients or residents diagnosed with dementia

- and who practises in accordance with a person-centred approach to care.

The rationale for eligibility was that the practice of nurses and allied healthcare practitioners focuses on the body as the primary site of their care work,[2] and it is precisely the physical nature of their clinical practice that provides them with the experience that is crucial to the body-based perspective on personhood that we wished to explore. Ethics approval was obtained by the ethics review boards of the participating study facilities.

Each focus group consisted of from six to eight practitioners at the given facility, with two focus groups conducted per facility. Forty-three practitioners, all of whom were female, participated: sixteen nurses, ten occupational therapists, eight physiotherapists, seven recreational therapists and two personal support workers.[3] Fewer personal support workers were recruited because two of the three facilities did not staff this category of practitioner. Participants were recruited from long-term care (67%), behavioural management units (26%) and geriatric rehabilitation (7%) units that varied in size (10-bed to 79-bed units) and resident/staff ratio (3:1 to 7:1).

Analysis
Focus group discussions were audio-recorded with the formal consent of participants. Verbatim transcripts were prepared for each focus group discussion and analysed using thematic analysis techniques (Denzin and Lincoln 1998). Descriptive coding was first conducted wherein segments of text were assigned a code reflecting the original statement. These codes then served as the basis for category formation. Categories with similar content were summarized, and ultimately these categories were further refined and formulated into fewer analytical categories through an inductive, iterative process of going back and forth between the data and our conceptual framework of embodied selfhood.

Results: Socio-cultural habits of the body
The data presented here[4] under the thematic category of 'socio-cultural habits of the body' capture how decision-making in the interpersonal moments of clinical practice is informed by practitioners' understanding of care recipients' socio-cultural bodily dispositions.

The importance of recognizing and responding positively to bodily modes of social expression by persons with dementia was discussed by focus group participants. For example, many participants recounted instances where residents' previous vocations instilled in them bodily dispositions to move and act in particular ways and, with some knowledge of the life history of those residents, the meaning of such expressions could be recognized. For example, a physiotherapist spoke of a resident who was a war veteran:

> There are a lot of war veterans who live here and I'll never forget this one resident who I worked with. I had a hell of a time getting him to stand up from his wheelchair so we could work on his walking... He refused. One day I was thinking about who this man was and what his life experiences were and started singing the national anthem. Well you wouldn't believe it but he stood up from his wheelchair and saluted me! So from then on we began our physio sessions with the national anthem.

Here the physiotherapist uses knowledge of the resident's previous vocation as a soldier to elicit from him an upright posture. She creatively uses the national anthem anticipating that as a soldier he would stand at attention. The immediate recognition of the anthem by the resident and his standing in salute of the physiotherapist powerfully illustrate how his previous vocation continues to be expressed in his bodily dispositions.

Socio-cultural bodily dispositions were described by practitioners as also observably manifest in residents' awareness of, and respect for, social conventions. In the following incident a nurse discovers that the source of a resident's resistance to morning care was his desire for privacy:

> I have a gentleman who always was resistive when I tried to remove his pants during care. He would keep pulling them back up or just push my hands away. So I took some time to speak to the wife to figure out what was happening, and she says he always was a very private man, always closing the bathroom door and covering himself when he would bathe. So I came up with the idea to attach Velcro to the towels we use so I could get his pants off without him being exposed. So we use that around him, you know, during care, and because you have him covered, he's less resistive, and it's much easier and less time-consuming to get his care done.

Similarly commenting on embodied expressions of social etiquette, a recreational therapist recounted the importance of hats for the residents of a veterans' facility:

> Hats. I find that hats, because I do a lot of outings, you know, it's like, 'oh, we got to wear a hat'. They're used to wearing a hat to go out, and then we enter a building, off comes the hat, you know. And I used to do a lot of Legion trips. If anyone wore a hat to go into a Legion, they had to buy everybody a round of beer. So you see, once they're coming in, oops, there

goes the hat, you know. So some of those things that they've grown up with or have done their whole life stay with them.

Awareness of, and respect for, such conventions can also be inferred from the reaction of some residents to other residents who fail to adhere to proper etiquette. As the same recreational therapist comments:

> I'm thinking of someone who when he was more mobile, he used to hit a lot of people in the dining room, and it was because they were wearing their hats at the table, but you don't wear a hat when you're sitting at the dining table. He would go in there and knock their hats off their heads.

Here the therapist recognized that the behaviour of those who did not remove their hats at the dining table was unacceptable for this particular resident and that his behaviour was thus a reaction to the other residents' violation of social etiquette. Her recognition of the meaning of the resident's actions led to her reassigning him to a table where no one wore a hat, successfully resolving the resident's aggressive outbursts in the dining room without needing to resort to other alternatives such as psychotropic medications.

Discussion

Our data indicate that there is a socio-cultural style or content to bodily movements and gestures, and that such socio-cultural self-expression informs in a significant way practitioners' decision-making regarding their approach to care. The social significance of the body is apparent in the focus group participants' discussion of their recognition of socio-cultural bodily dispositions of their care recipients. The data indicate that residents' tendencies and inclinations to move and behave in a particular manner were linked, for example, to their previous vocation, as with the resident who was previously a soldier. Practitioners also spoke of residents' awareness of, and respect for, social conventions, such as removing one's hat upon entering a Legion hall or before dining. These data indicate that social and cultural habits, movements and other physical cues disclose significant information about the particularity of the residents which brings the personhood of the residents into focus for the practitioners. This is consistent with Kontos' argument that 'selfhood [is] embodied and manifests in socio-culturally specific ways of being-in-the-world' (Kontos 2004, p.842). To articulate the socio-cultural sources of selfhood Kontos draws upon Bourdieu's notion of habitus, which foregrounds the socio-cultural sources of bodily habits. Bourdieu argues that the conditioning associated with socialization tends, through the relationship to one's own body, to instil in the

194 • DECISION-MAKING, PERSONHOOD AND DEMENTIA

individual dispositions and generative schemes for being and perceiving.[5] Bodily expressions (e.g. the ways in which we walk or eat) stress the durability of the effects of socialization through a cumulative exposure to certain social conditions associated with membership in a particular cultural group. Bourdieu defines a disposition as 'a *way of being*, a *habitual state*…a *tendency, propensity*, or *inclination*' (1977, p.214, n1, original emphasis). In the same way that dispositions are embodied and materialize as postures, gestures and movements (Bourdieu 1990), Kontos argues that selfhood is embodied and is manifested in 'our habitual state, tendencies and inclinations to act in a particular way' (2004, p.842).

Of paramount importance to the concept of habitus is the notion that an individual's actions are the product of a *modus operandi* of which the individual has no conscious mastery (Bourdieu 1977). This is aptly captured by Bourdieu in the following:

> …habitus…function[s]…as principles which generate and organize practices and representations that can be objectively adapted to their outcomes without presupposing a conscious aiming at ends or an express mastery of the operations necessary in order to attain them. Objectively 'regulated' and 'regular' without being in any way the product of obedience to rules, they can be collectively orchestrated without being the product of the organizing action of a conductor. (1990, p.53)

The pre-reflective nature of habitus is of critical importance to Kontos' articulation of selfhood in the context of Alzheimer's disease. Selfhood persists despite the presence and progression of Alzheimer's disease because it resides in the dispositions and generative schemes of habitus, below the threshold of cognition and in the pre-reflective level of experience (Kontos 2004).

Socio-cultural bodily dispositions are fundamental to practitioners' decision-making in that they disclose their care recipients' individuality, which facilitates the tailoring of care to accommodate their idiosyncrasies. The importance of having some understanding of the life history of another person for caring has been identified (Benhabib 1992; Hamington 2004; Mayeroff 1971). As Hamington, for example, argues, (2004, p.42), 'as the details and specific context of people become increasingly known…they become persons with names, faces, bodies, and other aspects to which sympathetic identification gives us a connection'. Mayeroff (1971) similarly argues that to care for someone requires having some knowledge of who they are and what their strengths and limitations are. Knowledge of another person as a critical ingredient for caring is also consistent with Benhabib's (1992) argument that caring arises from having knowledge of the particulars of the 'concrete other', their histories, attitudes, characters and desires. Our data too indicate that the impulse to care is bound up with knowledge of the care recipient. As the example of the resident resisting morning care indicates, as do the examples where residents' previous vocations instilled in them bodily dispositions to move and act in particular ways, under certain circumstances clearly some knowledge of life history is illuminating and facilitates the giving of care by rendering the resident's socio-cultural bodily dispositions recognizable to the practitioner.

Conclusion

Our data indicate that some practitioners are using knowledge of their care recipients' habits and practices to individualize their approach to care. More specifically, socio-cultural bodily dispositions disclose their care recipients' individuality, which provides the basis for clinical judgments that practitioners make about strategies for care. This is not to suggest that recognizing socio-cultural bodily dispositions alone is sufficient for decision-making around behavioural management. However, when acute physical illness and physical discomfort are excluded as triggers of aberrant behaviours, and when expressed personhood is identified as the trigger, it is significant that the appropriate tailoring of care has the potential to reduce these behaviours without the need to resort to psychotropic medications and other forms of restraint (Kontos and Naglie 2007a).

Our study indicates that there are care providers who are recognizing and supporting expressions of selfhood as they are manifest in care recipients' gestures and actions. Yet given that the quality of care in residential and nursing homes is in need of radical improvement (Ballard *et al.* 2001), clearly such humanistic caring practices are not systematically implemented across care settings (Ballard *et al.* 2001; Crawshaw 1996). Caring is a complex phenomenon. In order to further our understanding of this complexity, to grasp how to nurture the communicative capacity of the body, and what the optimal circumstances are for tailoring of care in accordance with this capacity, further qualitative inquiry is necessary. Qualitative methods can furnish descriptions and analyses that further explicate and inform our understanding of why some practitioners recognize embodied self-expressions that persist despite the ravages inflicted by neuropathology, and the ways in which such recognition facilitates person-centred approaches to care.

We are not suggesting that embodied selfhood alone should inform clinical decision-making in the practice of dementia care. We are, however, suggesting that embodied selfhood of persons with dementia provides an invaluable resource for decision-making that is integral to the provision of sympathetic dementia care. When we consider the possibilities that are presented by recognizing the importance of the body for self-expression, it is clear that we can no longer afford to ignore this vital source of selfhood that persists despite even severe cognitive impairment, but that has largely gone unrecognized. Our exploration of the communicative capacity of the body to connect practitioners to the personhood of their care recipients, thereby fostering sympathetic care, is intended to provide new insight and direction for future investigation of the body as an important resource for clinical decision-making.

ACKNOWLEDGMENTS

This study was generously funded by the Collaborative Research Program: Rehabilitation & Long-Term Care, the Canadian Nurses Foundation and the Nursing Care Partnership. The study was conducted during the tenure of Dr Kontos' postdoctoral fellowship that was supported by the Canadian Institutes of Health Research (CIHR) Fellowship Program (2004–2007; MFE-70433) and the Health Care, Technology, & Place CIHR Strategic Research & Training Program (2004–2007) (supported by CIHR Institutes of Health Services and Policy Research, Gender and Health, and Knowledge Translation Secretariat). Dr Kontos is presently supported by an Ontario Ministry of Health and Long-Term Care Career Scientist Award (2007–2012; #06388) that facilitated the writing of this chapter. Dr Naglie is supported by the Mary Trimmer Chair in Geriatric Medicine Research, University of Toronto. Toronto Rehabilitation Institute receives funding under the Provincial Rehabilitation Research Program from the Ministry of Health and Long-Term Care in Ontario. The views expressed here do not necessarily reflect those of our supporters or funders.

ENDNOTES

1. For a more detailed description of the methods employed in this study see Kontos and Naglie (2007a, 2007b).
2. Though physicians deal with the body, medical practice is constructed in such a way as to confine direct bodywork to the activity of diagnosis or to mediate it by high-tech machines (Twigg 2000). Recreational therapists were included given that in the activities they organize (exercise, music, social tea, etc.) they would have close proximity to residents that would provide them with opportunities to observe residents' bodily habits and gestures.

3.   In the focus groups where the personal support workers were present, there was no discernible power dynamic. All participants were fully engaged in the discussion and ideas and experiences were shared freely. We can only speculate that the participants' full commitment to the issue of person-centred dementia care rendered their status differences irrelevant.

4.   The findings of this study have received a more extensive elaboration elsewhere (Kontos and Naglie 2007a, 2007b).

5.   Our discussion here draws upon Kontos' articulation of Bourdieu's theory of the social and cultural dimensions of the body (2004, 2006a, 2006b).

REFERENCES

Andrews, G. (2006) 'Managing challenging behaviour in dementia.' *British Medical Journal* *332*, 7544, 741.

Ballard, C., Fossey, J., Chithramohan, R., Howard, R., *et al.* (2001) 'Quality of care in private sector and NHS facilities for people with dementia: Cross sectional survey.' *British Medical Journal 323*, 7310, 426–427.

Benhabib, S. (1992) *Situating the Self: Gender, Community and Postmodernism in Contemporary Ethics.* New York: Routledge.

Bourdieu, P. (1977) *Outline of a Theory of Practice.* Cambridge: Cambridge University Press.

Bourdieu, P. (1990) *The Logic of Practice.* Cambridge: Polity Press.

Bronskill, S.E., Anderson, G.M., Sykora, K., Wodchis, W.P. *et al* (2004) 'Neuroleptic drug therapy in older adults newly admitted to nursing homes: Incidence, dose, and specialist contact.' *Journal of the American Geriatrics Society 52*, 5, 749–755.

Chan, P. and Kenny, S.R. (2001) 'National consistency and provincial diversity in delivery of long-term care in Canada.' *Journal of Aging and Social Policy 13*, 2/3, 83–99.

Cohen-Mansfield, J. (1996) 'Conceptualization of agitation: Results based upon the Cohen-Mansfield agitation inventory and the Agitation Behaviour Mapping Instrument.' *International Psychogeriatrics 9*, 309–315.

Cohen-Mansfield, J. (2001) 'Nonpharmacologic interventions for inappropriate behaviors in dementia.' *American Journal of Geriatric Psychiatry 9*, 361–381.

Cohen-Mansfield, J. and Mintzer, J.E. (2005) 'Time for change: The role of nonpharmacological interventions in treating behavior problems in nursing home residents with dementia.' *Alzheimer Disease and Associated Disorders 19*, 1, 37–40.

Crawshaw, R. (1996) 'The cost of caring: A view of Britain's delivery of health care.' *Pharos*, Winter, 11–15.

DeDeyn, P.P., Rabheru, K., Rasmussen, A., Bocksberger, J.P. *et al.* (1999) 'A randomized trial of risperidone, placebo and haloperidol for behavioral symptoms of dementia.' *Neurology 53*, 5, 946–955.

Denzin, N.K. (2000) 'Aesthetics and the practices of qualitative inquiry.' *Qualitative Inquiry 6*, 2, 256–265.

Denzin, N.K. and Lincoln, Y.S. (1998) *Collecting and Interpreting Qualitative Materials.* Thousand Oaks, CA: Sage.

Dobbs, D., Munn, J., Zimmerman, S., Boustani, M. *et al.* (2005) 'Characteristics associated with lower activity involvement in long-term care residents with dementia.' *The Gerontologist 45*, 1, 81–86.

Douglas, S., James, I. and Ballard, C. (2004) 'Non-pharmacological interventions in dementia.' *Advances in Psychiatric Treatment 10*, 171–179.

Douzjian, M., Wilson, C. and Shultz, M. (1998) 'A program to use pain control medication to reduce psychotropic drug use in residents with difficult behavior.' *Annals of Long-Term Care 6*, 174–179.

Emerson, E. (1998) 'Working with People with Challenging Behaviour.' In E. Emerson, C. Hatton, A. Craine and J. Bromley (eds) *Clinical Psychology and People with Intellectual Disabilities.* Chichester: Wiley.

Fossey, J., Ballard, C., Juszczak, E., James, I. *et al.* (2006) 'Effect of enhanced psychosocial care on antipsychotic use in nursing home residents with severe dementia: Cluster randomised trial.' *British Medical Journal 332*, 7544, 756–761.

Geda, Y.E. and Rummans, T.A. (1999) 'Cause of agitation in elderly individuals with dementia.' *American Journal of Psychiatry 156*, 1662–1663.

Hall, L. and Kiesners, D. (2005) 'A narrative approach to understanding the nursing work environment in Canada.' *Social Science and Medicine 61*, 12, 2482–2491.

Hamers, J., Gulpers, M. and Strick, W. (2004) 'Use of physical restraints with cognitively impaired nursing home residents.' *Journal of Advanced Nursing 45*, 246–251.

Hamington, M. (2004) *Embodied Care: Jane Addams, Maurice Merleau-Ponty, and Feminist Ethics.* Urbana, IL: University of Illinois Press.

Henderson, J.A. and Vesperi, M.D. (1995) *The Culture of Long Term Care: Nursing Home Ethnography.* New York: Bergin and Garvey.

Hubbard, G., Cook, A., Tester, S. and Downs, M. (2002) 'Beyond words: Older people with dementia using and interpreting nonverbal behaviour.' *Journal of Aging Studies 16*, 155–167.

Kitwood, T. (1997) *Dementia Reconsidered: The Person Comes First.* Buckingham: Open University Press.

Kontos, P. (2004) 'Ethnographic reflections on selfhood, embodiment and Alzheimer's disease.' *Ageing and Society 24*, 829–849.

Kontos, P. (2005) 'Embodied selfhood in Alzheimer's disease: Rethinking person-centred care.' *Dementia 4*, 4, 553–570.

Kontos, P. (2006a) 'Embodied Selfhood: An Ethnographic Exploration of Alzheimer's Disease.' In L. Cohen and A. Leibing (eds) *Thinking about Dementia: Culture, Loss, and the Anthropology of Senility.* Cambridge: Cambridge University Press.

Kontos, P. (2006b) 'Habitus: An incomplete account of human agency.' *American Journal of Semiotics 22*, 67–83.

Kontos, P. and Naglie, G. (2006) 'Expressions of personhood in Alzheimer's: Moving from ethnographic text to performing ethnography.' *Qualitative Research 6*, 3, 301–317.

Kontos, P. and Naglie, G. (2007a) 'Bridging theory and practice: Imagination, the body, and person-centred dementia care.' *Dementia 6*, 4, 549–569.

Kontos, P. and Naglie, G. (2007b) 'Expressions of personhood in Alzheimer's disease: An evaluation of research-based theatre as a pedagogical tool.' *Qualitative Health Research 17*, 6, 799–811.

Kovach, C.R., Taneli, Y., Dohearty, P., Schlidt, A.M., Cashin, S. and Silva-Smith, A.L. (2004) 'Effect of the BACE intervention on agitation of people with dementia.' *The Gerontologist 44*, 6, 797–806.

Margallo-Lana, M., Swann, A., O'Brien, J., Fairbairn, A. *et al.* (2001) 'Prevalence and pharmacological management of behavioural and psychological symptoms amongst dementia sufferers living in care environments.' *International Journal of Geriatric Psychiatry 16*, 1, 39–44.

Mark, B. (2002) 'What explains nurses' perceptions of staffing adequacy?' *Journal of Nursing Administration 32*, 5, 234–242.

Mayeroff, M. (1971) *On Caring*. New York: Harper and Row.

McCormack, B. (2004) 'Person-centredness in gerontological nursing: An overview of the literature.' *International Journal of Older People Nursing 13*, 3a, 31–38.

Moniz-Cook, E., Woods, R.T. and Richards, K. (2001) 'Functional analysis of challenging behaviour in dementia: The role of superstition.' *International Journal of Geriatric Psychiatry 16*, 45–56.

Nolan, M.R., Booth, A. and Nolan, J. (1997) *New Directions in Rehabilitation: Exploring the Nursing Contribution*. London: English National Board for Nursing, Midwifery and Health Visiting.

Rader, J., Barrick, A.L., Hoeffer, B., Sloane, P.D. *et al.* (2006) 'The bathing of older adults with dementia.' *American Journal of Nursing 106*, 4, 40–48.

Rochon, P.A., Stukel, T.A., Bronskill, S.E., Gomes, T. *et al.* (2007) 'Variation in nursing home antipsychotic prescribing rates.' *Archives of Internal Medicine 167*, 7, 676–683.

Sink, K.M., Holden, K.F. and Yaffe, K. (2005) 'Pharmacological treatment of neuropsychiatric symptoms of dementia: A review of evidence.' *Journal of the American Medical Association 293*, 596–608.

Stokes, G. (1996) 'Challenging Behavior in Dementia: A Psychological Approach.' In R.T. Woods (ed.) *Handbook of the Clinical Psychology of Ageing*. Chicester: Wiley.

Street, J.S., Clark, W.S., Gannon, K.S., Cummings, J.L. *et al.* (2000) 'Olanzapine treatment of psychotic and behavioral symptoms in patients with Alzheimer disease in nursing care facilities: A double-blind randomized, placebo-controlled trial.' *Archives of General Psychiatry 57*, 968–976.

Twigg, J. (2000) *Bathing: The Body and Community Care*. London: Routledge.

Whittemore, R. (2000) 'Consequences of not "knowing the patient".' *Clinical Nurse Specialist 14*, 2, 75–81.

Conclusion

CHAPTER 15

Decision-Making and Dementia
Toward a Social Model of Understanding

DEBORAH O'CONNOR, BARBARA PURVES AND
MURNA DOWNS

This book, *Decision-Making, Personhood and Dementia: Exploring the Interface*,
addresses the implications of a social constructionist view of personhood in
dementia for practice and research around decision-making. A social constructionist perspective challenges essentialist ideas about dementia, proposing
instead a more fluid and contextual response that is shaped by one's interactions with one's world. The purpose of this volume was to examine how this
approach could complement and extend the more clinically based health and
legal literature that currently grounds understanding in this area. The chapters
in the volume represent a multi-disciplinary approach to this exploration,
emphasizing the complexity and importance of context to research and
practice in this area. This final chapter identifies four interrelated themes that
emerge across the chapters taken as a whole:

- Deconstructing autonomy: Interrogating the notion of a
  self-determining individual

- Reconceptualizing decision-making: Implications of a relational
  approach

- Broadening the focus: Developing and using a person-centred
  assessment of capacity

- Redirecting attention: Empowerment and maximizing participation.

These overlapping themes point to two key messages. The first is the requirement to challenge a conventional focus on autonomy that prioritizes the cognitively capable individual, proposing instead the importance of a relational understanding. The second message reflects the importance of shifting the focus in discussions about decision-making from concerns with establishing individual capacity and competence to a more inclusive understanding of the person's perspective and retained strengths, thus maximizing participation irrespective of cognitive functioning. Combined, these messages suggest the importance of moving toward a social model for understanding decision-making in dementia.

DECONSTRUCTING AUTONOMY: INTERROGATING THE NOTION OF A SELF-DETERMINING INDIVIDUAL

Deconstructing involves challenging accepted ways of understanding the world that are often taken as 'givens'. Deconstructing these givens involves examining and interrogating them in relation to their social, historical and political contexts (O'Connor 2003). The intent is to disrupt seemingly smooth social surfaces and accepted wisdom in order to create the space for alternative discourses. Most of the chapters in this volume challenge the privileged position of autonomy, arguing that it has been conventionally understood in relation to individualism within the decision-making process. Either explicitly or implicitly, the importance of deconstructing this notion of autonomy is raised. Within most discussions on decision-making, the focus on autonomy is rarely deconstructed or challenged and its value is accepted as a given. As demonstrated by several of the papers in this book, adopting a social constructionist view of personhood leads to challenging individualist and cognitive-based notions of autonomy.

Discussions about decision-making have traditionally been influenced by principle-based biomedical ethics that promote autonomy as one of four guiding principles. Autonomy is the right to self-determination, and it provides the foundation for considerations around capacity and competence. This principle along with beneficence (do good), justice (be fair) and non-maleficence (do no harm) comprise the four principles of ethical decision-making frameworks (see for example Beauchamp and Childress 1994). In these frameworks autonomy and beneficence (including the concept of protection of another's best interests) are often discussed as being in opposition to one another. By dichotomizing these two concepts – autonomy and beneficence – the implication is that autonomy stands apart from protection, and is unquestionably the dominant ideal. In this book autonomy is challenged on a variety of grounds:

- it is far from being a universal discourse
- it disadvantages those for whom it is less meaningful or central
- it neglects the social and interpersonal context in which individuals lead their lives and make decisions.

First and foremost, this book challenges the principle of autonomy as a universal discourse, or story-line, for organizing people's actions and behaviours. For example, Tsai (Chapter 5) highlights the inadequacy of this notion within Eastern culture for defining personhood; he draws on Confucianism to outline a more relational approach for guiding decision-making in relation to the care of persons with dementia that is more congruent with Eastern values. Similarly, assumptions about the primacy of autonomy-based values to guide practices around understanding capacity and the decision-making process are recognized as potentially disadvantaging both women (O'Connor and Donnelly, Chapter 8) and people from other cultural groups (Hulko and Stern, Chapter 6).

Autonomy then is exposed as a dominant Western ideal that has more – or less – meaning in the lives of people with dementia depending upon the socio-cultural context in which they are positioned. The implication for this in practice is that it opens to question the rationale being used to understand how people make decisions, including what constitutes a 'reasonable' decision and what practices are being used to guide substitute decision-makers. It highlights the ease with which those from non-dominant cultures may be pejoratively judged. Ultimately, it reinforces imperatives that healthcare professionals reflect upon how they are using their own value systems to judge situations if they are to be truly open to person-centred care practices.

Second, it leads us to ask: How does the focus on autonomy, as defined through dominant Western culture, benefit some to the detriment of others? From a research and conceptual perspective, deconstructing notions of autonomy in decision-making opens up new and important areas for development. Specifically, it is not sufficient to simply challenge autonomy as necessarily a universally prioritized discourse. Rather, discourses represent socio-political interests, and an important part of deconstructing a discourse is to examine how it is being used to establish and perpetuate power relations (Weedon 1987). Smith (Chapter 3) is most overt in promoting the need to consider this. He calls for a more contextualized reflection in relation to the social practices that define the nature of autonomy and decision-making practices, suggesting that, through the process of interrogating individualizing notions such as autonomy, it becomes clearer how particular approaches can legitimize oppressive practices that further negate the social existence of individuals with dementia. Specifically, he recognizes that this lens of autonomy-based decision-making may benefit some at the expense of others; in this situation, the 'other' is the person with dementia.

The third but closely linked point is that deconstructing autonomy opens our minds to the social and interpersonal context in which individuals lead their lives and make decisions. An important goal here is to begin to understand how individual everyday experiences are shaped by broader societal contexts. This agenda reflects the growing recognition that person-centred lenses must be extended to address the general issues of stigma and discrimination that confront people with dementia on a daily basis (see for example Baldwin 2008; Bartlett and O'Connor 2007). Employing the language of citizenship, the call is to move beyond the focus on the individual to examine collective experiences, including rights and responsibilities. Stephen Post (2000), in drawing attention to our hypercognitive society, has been influential in beginning to develop a broader socio-political context for understanding the devastation that may accompany the removal, or curtailment, of one's rights to autonomous decision-making and practice. Smith (Chapter 3) draws on the ideas of Pierre Bourdieu to suggest one way to extend this analysis. The point here is that there is an implicit link between cognition and individualism that underpins notions of conventional autonomy which will be important to tease out at a broader, structural level.

Little of the research focused on decision-making and dementia draws on this type of a critical lens. These are new ways of thinking about the place of autonomy (and arguably cognition) both within our society, but especially in the lives of persons with dementia. They require further development, understanding and implementation. Hence, the task of deconstructing autonomy can be seen as an important first step toward re-envisioning personhood, potentially providing a more useful framework for ethical decision-making. It may also provide a strategy to render visible how people with dementia are constructed as 'less than' within dominant Western society – at a minimum it names one of the processes through which this occurs.

How does this extend understanding related to dementia, personhood and decision-making? First, it suggests that health professionals must be careful about imposing a value system for understanding and evaluating decision-making that is implicitly premised on assumptions that everyone is motivated to be primarily independent autonomous beings. Second, it challenges society to think differently about taken-for-granted assumptions in order to query how they may be used to disadvantage some. In this situation, autonomy is equated with independence and capacity as the preferred, default position. To be dependent and incapable of making a decision necessarily positions the person with dementia in an inferior position. A way forward will require challenging this dichotomy as overly simplistic – neglecting for example the possibilities of interdependencies – as a step toward confronting the stigma and marginalization that are associated with dementia.

RECONCEPTUALIZING DECISION-MAKING: IMPLICATIONS OF A RELATIONAL APPROACH

In tandem with challenging the focus on autonomy, many of the chapters in this book propose an alternative, more relational-based approach to understanding decision-making, one that recognizes it as a dynamic interplay that takes place within an interpersonal and social context. This call resonates with a growing trend in healthcare ethics to challenge the principlism of normative ethics as a universal, or even as the best, approach to guide decision-making. This importance given to relationship in ethical decision-making has emerged in the last 20 years as an evolving concept with care-based ethics highlighting relationship as central to care (Gilligan 1982), feminist ethics emphasizing power relations (Sherwin 1992) and relational ethics promoting a central theme of connectedness in which 'we attend to the moral space created by one's relationship to oneself and to the other' (Bergum 2004, p.486). These approaches to ethical decision-making are consistent with a personhood approach that posits a relational, or social constructionist, lens for understanding and action.

Such an approach is concerned with the complexity associated with the decision-making process in dementia, seeing it as essentially dynamic, relational and context dependent. There are a number of ways that this theme of relational-based decision-making emerges in these chapters. For example, in the realm of policy and practice, O'Connor and Donnelly (Chapter 8) emphasize the importance of considering power relations in capacity assessments. Further, they make the case that women's decision-making can only be understood as 'reasonable' if a relational framework is applied. This point also emerges in Chapter 10, where Tilse, Wilson and Setterlund note that in their research older people commonly identified the importance of managing their assets within the context of family relationships, often expressing the desire to prioritize the maintenance of relationships over the quality of asset management being provided.

These findings highlight the need for formal assessments to allow for more nuanced and contextualized interpretations that take into account relational considerations. In circumstances where decision-making necessarily focuses on an individual, at the very least we should extend the notion of autonomy to that of relational autonomy, which Sherwin (1998) defined as 'a capacity or skill that is developed (and constrained) by social circumstances. It is exercised within relationships and social structures that jointly help to shape the individual while also affecting others' responses to her efforts at autonomy' (p.36). We will return to this point later in the chapter.

The focus on relational-based decision-making is particularly evident in chapters exploring everyday decision-making. This suggests that, in everyday life, individuals do tend to make decisions in the context of their relationships; however much we may be constructed as autonomous beings in social policy and practice, we nonetheless live our lives as relational beings. This hypothesis problematizes the intersection of public and private decision-making processes by highlighting crucial differences in their underlying assumptions about the relative importance of different stakeholders' contributions and needs. Specifically, O'Connor and Kelson's work (Chapter 12) draws attention to how one partner's needs can be subjugated to those of the other in accessing support services, raising the question of who the client is. Purves and Perry (Chapter 13) highlight how tensions between the widely accepted concepts of autonomy and protection are reinterpreted and enacted within a family, inviting exploration of how the public discourse of dementia influences understandings of what it means to have dementia and the implications for everyday decision-making. Finally, Kontos and Naglie (Chapter 14) question why only some carers use embodied selfhood – a central theme in Bergum's (2004) description of relational ethics – as a resource in dementia care; in doing so, they point to the need for further exploration of how organizational practices constrain relational approaches to care. This is a topic that Harrigan and Gillett also address at a broader conceptual level in their discussion of influences of modernity in Chapter 4.

Combining the first two themes then, one message that dominates across the chapters in this volume speaks to the importance of re-examining the principles that are being used to understand decision-making in order to ensure a focus away from individualism to a process that is more relationally focused. One practical implication of this shift is to recognize that one can neither understand nor deal with the person with dementia in isolation from his or her context. This is not a new message. But what has been less well articulated is the notion that, when taking a relational lens, the focus shifts from the individual, per se, to the relationship. This introduces messiness to decision-making that requires far more consideration.

BROADENING THE FOCUS: DEVELOPING AND USING A PERSON-CENTRED ASSESSMENT OF CAPACITY

At the core of any discussion on decision-making is the convergence of attention to concepts of capacity and competence. Particularly in the clinical health and legal literatures this is highlighted as a critical area for exploration and development. Unquestionably it is important to improve understanding of issues associated with assessing capacity and competence. Legally removing someone's rights to direct one's own life, or aspects of it, may be a dramatic, powerful and potentially devastating action. Hence, finding ways to evaluate capacity that ensure increased reliability and validity is identified as high priority within the clinical health and legal literatures.

Interestingly, this series of papers does not foreground the assessment of capacity with the same level of significance or intensity as can be found in the clinical health and legal literatures. With few exceptions, these papers do not explicitly address the actual assessment process, nor do they draw attention to the lack of assessment tools. Indirectly, however, many do offer insights into the development and use of capacity assessments. In particular, four relevant ideas can be identified: the first regards what is being assessed, the second raises questions regarding how the assessment should be accomplished, the third addresses the inextricable link between the process of assessing and the outcome of the assessment, and the fourth recognizes the limitations associated with a focus on capacity.

First, what is being assessed? At the simplest level, an approach to decision-making that is grounded in an understanding of personhood demands a more person-centred assessment of capacity. This idea is consistent with concerns being raised in the clinical health and legal literatures. Specifically, there has been widespread criticism that, too frequently, assessments of capacity have been overly focused upon cognition at the expense of a more holistic understanding. (See for example O'Connor and Donnelly, Chapter 8, this volume, or Kluge 2005, for a review and discussion of this issue.) Within the more conventional clinical health and legal literatures, the need to broaden the focus to include attention to both emotional context and values has been identified. Certainly the chapters in this volume would support this, suggesting that cognition cannot stand in isolation of the entire person.

The second issue regards the 'how' of assessing. The clinical health and legal literatures emphasize the need for better strategies for conducting assessments. Often this translates into the language of better 'tools'. While the congruence of a standardized tool with a personhood approach seems tantamount to an oxymoron, newer conceptual models that are more person-centred are beginning to emerge. For example, Moye and colleagues (2007) propose a conceptual model and assessment template that is structured around six domains:

medical condition, cognition, functional abilities, values, risk of harm and level of supervision needed, and means to enhance capacity. Ideally, this approach lends itself to a more person-centred assessment. However, there is concern that, historically, these tools have been appropriated and used in a way that counters person-centredness and perhaps even perpetrates oppressive practices. Smith (Chapter 3), for example, recognizes that there are non-altruistic motives behind the quest to develop assessment tools. Exploring who benefits and how opens up new ways for understanding and using standardized tools. This critical perspective leads to thought-provoking questions including: How do assessments of capacity normalize the process by which persons with dementia become marginalized? What does the field stand to gain by integrating more standardized tools? What does it lose?

Furthermore, countering the priority of attention to developing standardized tools, several chapters draw on the importance of the narrative turn as a more apposite means for improving the assessment process. Most explicitly, Baldwin (Chapter 2) provides the conceptual foundation for understanding the importance of a shift toward narrative decision-making while Keady, Williams and Hughes-Roberts (Chapter 11) apply this lens to demonstrate how four people's actions around the decision to seek diagnosis can best be understood when contextualized within their broader story. Suggested here is that there may be a place for tools to supplement understanding, but that these tools will always be an inferior way of hearing the whole story. Rather, the basic and fundamental practice of listening to what people say – and how they say it – remains the critical process for understanding how someone with dementia is making a decision.

While the what and the how have been discussed as though they were separate aspects of the assessment, a third point that emerges quite clearly when drawing on social constructionist notions of personhood is that these two are, in fact, inextricably linked. Although the importance of creating a therapeutic assessment context is certainly recognized in more conventional literature, it is much more clearly conceptualized when drawing on social constructionist ideas. Specifically, if one's performances and self-perceptions – indeed one's sense of self as a unique person – are constructed within one's relational contexts, there should be an assumption that cognition will fluctuate depending upon how the person is treated and understood. Thus, the importance of establishing a respectful relationship and practices that foster a sense of competence becomes pivotal. As Sabat (2005) notes:

...when others refuse to cooperate with the person with AD in the construction of a valued social identity, the person is restricted to the identity of 'dysfunctional patient' and any 'loss of self' has its roots in the social world rather than the brain of the person in question. (p.1034)

The implications of this point are twofold: the assessment must be more holistic and affirming, and findings related to capacity must be recognized as potentially fluid and dependent upon the context.

The fourth issue related to capacity is the need to recognize the limitations associated with narrowly restricting the focus on decision-making to the issue of capacity. Certainly the research presented in this volume examining decision-making in everyday living suggests that incapacity may take a distant backseat to other considerations, particularly those linked to maintaining meaningful relationships. The emphasis upon capacity may not be the most relevant element of the decision-making process to persons with dementia and their families. Thus, a directive that cuts across many of the chapters in this volume is the need to expand beyond the focus on capacity to a broader discussion about decision-making. This challenge is indirectly taken up by most of the contributions in the third section, which focus on understanding decision-making in day-to-day activities. These chapters demonstrate how decision-making that promotes personhood occurs across a gamut of settings, even when the person with dementia is, arguably, 'incapable'.

The implication of this for practice is that health professionals must be attuned to a multiplicity of factors that are influencing the decisions being made – these may carry more weight than whether or not the person with dementia is actually 'capable' or not. In particular, within the familial relationship, more emphasis may be placed on facilitating a positive experience of one's self for the person with dementia than on challenging abilities. This point links back to the notion of a relational understanding and may be a particularly important area in which to probe further. Moreover, although it is often recognized that it is the decision-making process and not the decision itself that is being evaluated, few actually look beyond the determination of capacity to the actual decision-making process. There is concern that the focus on assessment has overshadowed attention to process. This point will be picked up in the following section.

REDIRECTING ATTENTION: EMPOWERMENT AND MAXIMIZING PARTICIPATION

Underpinning a number of the chapters in this volume is an interesting shift away from a focus on loss toward one of empowerment. This is not to downplay the importance of cognitive changes, but rather represents an attempt at rebalancing. Thus, in lieu of the autonomy/protection debate, the discussion appears to be broadening to include dual threads of empowerment and protection – these are presented as a continuum, rather than resorting to the classical split that occurs with discussions around autonomy and protection. Evidence of this shift is apparent in England's Mental Capacity Act 2005, where the need to begin to disentangle notions of autonomy from capacity is clearly recognized and where others are mandated to maximize participation in decisions even when it is clear that the person may lack capacity to actually make this decision (Manthorpe, Chapter 7, this volume; see also Boyle 2008). Tilse and her colleagues (Chapter 10) suggest a similar refocusing within the Australian context with regard to asset management. They note that this shift toward an empowerment model can be seen in discussions about 'assisted' decision-making as opposed to 'substitute' decision-making with the corresponding focus on making decisions with, and not for, people with dementia.

This focus on empowerment has the potential to offer important directions for moving discussions about decision-making to new levels that are more congruent with a personhood approach. For example, it challenges dichotomous thinking about capacity (is he or she capable or not?) by introducing a more nuanced focus that is individualized and process-oriented: How can this person be best involved? The trend toward a more complex understanding is consistent with the clinical health and legal literatures, where the focus on general competence has moved to decision-specific capacities that are recognized as situational. Drawing on notions of empowerment, the question of capacity is diverted still further from the standard 'Is he or she capable of this specific decision or action?' to 'How can he or she be involved irrespective of whether or not capacity is demonstrated?' This is particularly pertinent for people with dementia where cognitive functioning can at some point be expected to interfere with capacity in the conventional sense. The underlying assumption is that people with dementia can still be involved in decision-making even if cognitively they experience limiting problems that result in their being deemed 'incapable'.

Bringing in the notion of empowerment, then, introduces a more process-oriented understanding that begins to balance the negativity associated with the assessment of decisional capacity with a strength-based assessment. The focus shifts from a discrete determination of capacity to maximizing participation irrespective of capacity. Making this shift requires a holistic understanding of the person that takes into account that person's particular strengths and capabilities. Arguably, this will counter more deficit-based biomedical approaches, promoting a focus that is grounded by attention to personhood and not the disease process. In taking this approach, a social context is established that is more respectful and inclusive of people with dementia.

In a variety of ways, a number of the chapters pick up on this trend as an important area for practice and research development. Moreover, as Manthorpe (Chapter 7) demonstrates, it is clearly already happening within legislation. From a practice perspective, it appears that health and social care professionals will increasingly be challenged to see beyond determinations about decisional capacity to find real ways to include people with dementia in decisions that impact them. This epitomizes an approach to decision-making that draws on social constructionist notions of personhood.

How this will be accomplished remains an area for further exploration. Understanding and employing more effective communication strategies with people with dementia has been targeted as one means for facilitating inclusion within the personhood literature, but within the more conventional clinical health and legal literatures it has received less attention. Chapters in this volume (see for example Purves and Perry, Chapter 13; Kontos and Naglie, Chapter 14) extend this discussion to consider how day-to-day use of language, verbal and non-verbal, can promote inclusive – or exclusive – practices for involving people with dementia in decisions about their lives. In light of a shift toward developing more empowering practices around inclusion, this will be an important area to continue to develop.

Maximizing participation through individualizing strategies, such as strength-based assessments and modifying communication patterns, is critical. However, the importance of thinking creatively about empowerment is not limited to direct interactions with the person with dementia. Rather, there may be interesting and creative ways to use systems interventions to achieve this same goal. Hall (Chapter 9), for example, identifies how assessments of capacity can be bypassed entirely by drawing on legal doctrines of undue influence and unconscionability. She argues that these doctrines promote the shift in focus from an individual attribute (or deficit) to the characteristics of the situation. This work begins to hint at the importance of exploring structural changes and ways of making situations and contexts work better for people with dementia.

A focus on maximizing participation encapsulates the essence of an approach that is grounded by an understanding of personhood that is socially constructed within and by one's social context. It shifts the balance toward a more holistic, inspiring and healthy understanding of the dementia experience.

To conclude, introducing the notion of a socially constructed personhood into the debates and discussions around decision-making within a context of dementia moves forward understanding and actions in four important and interrelated ways. First, it draws attention to the limitations imposed by drawing upon an individualized notion of autonomy for directing practice.

Instead, it recognizes the person with dementia as interdependent and relationally bounded, comprehensible only within a context of social relationships. The second point then is that a relational understanding may offer an ecologically valid and more helpful way of understanding issues associated with decision-making. Third, when a more holistic and contextual approach is taken, notions of competence must extend beyond the focus on cognitive capacity to consider the links between behaviour, self-perception and societal treatment. Finally, shifting from a preoccupation with capacity to consider other aspects of the process, namely how to promote participation, provides the route toward an empowerment-oriented journey.

REFERENCES

Baldwin, C. (2008) 'Narrative, citizenship and dementia: The personal and the political.' *Journal of Aging Studies 22*, 222–228.

Bartlett, R. and O'Connor, D. (2007) 'From personhood to citizenship: Broadening the lens for dementia practice and research.' *Journal of Aging Studies 21*, 107–118.

Beauchamp, T.L. and Childress, J.F. (1994) *Principles of Biomedical Ethics* (4th edn). New York: Oxford University Press.

Bergum, V. (2004) 'Relational Ethics in Nursing.' In J.L. Storch, P. Rodney and R. Starzomski (eds) *Toward a Moral Horizon*. Toronto: Pearson Prentice-Hall.

Boyle, G. (2008) 'The Mental Capacity Act 2005: Promoting the citizenship of people with dementia?' *Health and Social Care in the Community 16*, 5, 529–537.

Gilligan, C. (1982) *In a Different Voice: Psychological Theory and Women's Development*. Cambridge, MA: Harvard University Press.

Kluge, E.H.W. (2005) 'Competence, capacity, and informed consent: Beyond the cognitive-competence model.' *Canadian Journal on Aging 24*, 3, 295–304.

Moye, J., Butz, S.W., Marson, D.C., Wood, E. and the ABA-APA Capacity Assessment of Older Adults Working Group (2007) 'A conceptual model and assessment template for capacity evaluation in adult guardianship.' *Gerontologist 47*, 5, 591–603.

O'Connor, D. (2003) 'Anti-Oppressive Practice in Older Adults: A Feminist, Post-Structural Perspective.' In W. Shearer (ed.) *Critical Perspectives on Anti-Oppressive Practice*. Toronto: Canadian Scholars Press.

Post, S.G. (2000) 'The Concept of Alzheimer Disease in a Hypercognitive Society.' In P.J. Whitehouse, K. Maurer and J.F. Ballenger (eds) *Concepts of Alzheimer Disease: Biological, Clinical, and Cultural Perspectives*. Baltimore, MD: Johns Hopkins University Press.

Sabat, S. (2005) 'Capacity for decision-making in Alzheimer's disease: Selfhood, positioning and semiotic people.' *Australian and New Zealand Journal of Psychiatry 39*, 11–12, 1030–1035.

Sherwin, S. (1992) *No Longer Patient: Feminist Ethics and Health Care*. Philadelphia: Temple University Press.

Sherwin, S. (1998) 'A Relational Approach to Autonomy in Health Care.' In S. Sherwin and The Feminist Health Care Ethics Research Network (eds) *The Politics of Women's Health: Exploring Agency and Autonomy*. Philadelphia: Temple University Press.

Weedon, C. (1987) *Feminist Practice and Poststructuralist Theory*. New York: Basil Blackwell.

Contributors

Clive Baldwin is a senior lecturer in the Bradford Dementia Group, University of Bradford, UK. He also holds a faculty position in the Department of Social Work, University of Bradford.

Martha Donnelly is Director, Division of Community Geriatrics, Department of Family Practice, and Division of Geriatric Psychiatry, Department of Psychiatry, University of British Columbia. She is a geriatric psychiatrist in Vancouver, BC, and a researcher with the Centre for Research on Personhood in Dementia at the University of British Columbia in Vancouver.

Murna Downs holds the positions of Chair in Dementia Studies and Head, Bradford Dementia Group, University of Bradford, UK.

Grant Gillett is a neurosurgeon and Professor of Medical Ethics, Dunedin Hospital and Otago Bioethics Centre, University of Otago Medical School, Dunedin, New Zealand.

Margaret Isabel Hall is a lawyer who has taught law at the University of British Columbia, the University of Ottawa and the University of Saskatchewan (the Native Law Centre). She is also a research associate at the Centre for Research on Personhood in Dementia at the University of British Columbia in Vancouver, BC.

MaryLou Harrigan is a healthcare consultant and educator in Vancouver, British Columbia. She recently completed a post-doctoral fellowship with the Centre for Research on Personhood in Dementia at the University of British Columbia in Vancouver, BC.

John Hughes-Roberts is a clinical nurse specialist in the Division of Mental Health and Disability, Conwy and Denbighshire NHS Trust, Glan Traeth Day Hospital, Wales.

Wendy Hulko is an assistant professor in the Social Work at Thompson Rivers University, Kamloops, BC, and a researcher with the Centre for Research on Personhood in Dementia at the University of British Columbia in Vancouver, BC.

John Keady is Professor of Older People's Mental Health Nursing in the School of Nursing, Midwifery and Social Work, University of Manchester. He is also co-editor of *Dementia: The International Journal of Social Research and Practice.*

Elizabeth Kelson is a research assistant and doctoral fellow in the Centre for Research on Personhood in Dementia at the University of British Columbia in Vancouver, BC. She is currently taking a PhD in Interdisciplinary Studies.

Pia C. Kontos is a research scientist at Toronto Rehabilitation Institute and Assistant Professor at the Dalla Lana School of Public Health, University of Toronto, Canada.

Jill Manthorpe is Professor of Social Work and Director of the Social Care Workforce Research Unit at King's College London, UK.

Gary Naglie is a consultant geriatrician and senior scientist at Toronto Rehabilitation Institute and University Health Network. He is also the Mary Trimmer Chair in Geriatric Medicine Research and associate professor in the Departments of Medicine and Health Policy, Management and Evaluation, University of Toronto, Canada.

Deborah O'Connor is the Director of the Centre for Research on Personhood in Dementia and an associate professor in the School of Social Work at the University of British Columbia in Vancouver, BC.

JoAnn Perry is Professor Emeritus, School of Nursing, University of British Columbia. She is also a researcher with the Centre for Research on Personhood in Dementia at the University of British Columbia in Vancouver, BC.

Barbara Purves is an assistant professor in the School of Audiology and Speech Sciences, University of British Columbia. She is also a researcher with the Centre for Research on Personhood in Dementia at the University of British Columbia in Vancouver, BC.

Deborah Setterlund is a social worker and adjunct senior lecturer in the School of Social Work and Human Services, University of Queensland, Australia.

André Smith is an assistant professor in the Department of Sociology, University of Victoria, British Columbia. He is an associate researcher with the Centre for Research on Personhood in Dementia at the University of British Columbia in Vancouver, BC.

Louise Stern is a social worker at Louis Brier Home and Hospital. She is a sessional instructor in the School of Social Work, University of British Columbia, and a doctoral fellow with the Centre for Research on Personhood in Dementia at the University of British Columbia in Vancouver, BC.

Cheryl Tilse is an associate professor in the School of Social Work and Human Services at the University of Queensland, Australia. She is a chief investigator of the Assets and Ageing research team.

Daniel Fu-Chang Tsai is the Acting Director, Center for Ethics, Law and Society in Biomedicine & Technology, at the National Taiwan University. He also holds a post as Associate Professor, Department of Social Medicine at the National Taiwan University College of Medicine and Attending Physician, Department of Medical Research at the National Taiwan University Hospital.

Sion Williams is a lecturer in the School of Nursing, Midwifery and Health Studies, University of Wales, Bangor.

Jill Wilson holds the Uniting Care Chair, Social Policy and Research in the School of Social Work and Human Services at the University of Queensland, a position that seeks to promote research in that large voluntary organization and to contribute to policy debates in a range of areas, including issues affecting older people.

Subject Index

abilities/inabilities, assumptions of 180
Adult Guardianship Act (AGA) 2000 (British Columbia) 100, 110
adult protection 100
Adults and Incapacity Act 2000 (Scotland) 93
advance decisions 99
advanced dementia 19
advocacy 101
age, and undue influence 127, 129–30
agency 38, 140
aggressive treatments 59
agitation management 187–8
Alice 77–8
altruism 63
Alzheimer's Disease (AD) 148, 150–4, 160
    family case study 175–84
Alzheimer's Disease (AD) study 149–50
    bridging 150–7
assessments
    appropriateness for use 112
    clinical practice 18
    conceptual models 209–10
    context-dependency 208
    formal 11
    retrospective 121–3
    standardized tools 210
    symbolic violence of 42–4
    see also capacity assessment
asset managers 137–8
assets 133–5, 138, 139, 140–1, 207, 212
Assets and Ageing research program 135–42
attorneys 97
autonomy 12, 17, 60–1, 63, 71
    as basis of decision-making 74–5
    capacity assessment 115
    deconstructing 204–7
    differential benefits of focus on 205–6

limitations of focus 213–14
    and personhood 73–4
    relational perspective 204
    self-directed support 94
Avon v. Bridger, [1985] 2 All ER 281 (CA) 127–8
Away From Her 54

Barclays Bank v. O'Brien, [1994] 1 AC180 (HL) 127–8
behaviour, interventions 187–8
beneficence 204–5
bioethics 60–1, 66–7, 78–81
Black v. Wilcox (1976), 12 OR (2d) 759 (CA) 129
body 188–9, 193–4, 195, 196
    see also focus group study: embodied selfhood
Bridger v. Bridger 2005 BCSC 269 120–1
bridging 150–7
bureaucracy 50

Calumsky v. Karaloff, [1946] SCR 110 128
Calvert v. Calvert (1997), 32 OR (3d) 281 121–3
capable but vulnerable 119
capacity 120–1
    bypassing 110
    as criterion of personhood 60–1, 66
    decision-making 131
    decision-specific 212
    defining 11–12
    domains 110
    equity theory 124–31
    in everyday living 15–16
    focus on 211
    importance of context 107
    informal appraisals 140–1
    not key issue 204
    person-centred assessment 209–12
    standards for evaluation 110–11

capacity assessment 12, 37, 96, 110–12
    dimensions of 137
    disempowerment 113–16
    elder abuse 112–16
    focus on cognition 209
    gendered understanding 115–16
    person-centred 209–12
    power relations 114
    predictive 123–4
    retrospective 121–3
    safety issues 112–13
care, social model 13–15
carers 96, 165
Carys 150, 151, 152, 153–4, 154–5
Centre for Research on Personhood in Dementia (CRPD) 17
character 33–4, 55
character and role 28–9
choices 95, 102
chun-tze 63–6
Chung-yung 65
class structure 38–9
clinical assessment practices, symbolic violence of 42–4
clinical practice, assessments 18
codes of ethics 73
coherency and consistency, of narrative 31–2
collectivism 42, 74–81
comedy 27
Commercial Bank of Australia v. Amadio (1983), 151 CLR 461 128–9
commitments, reflected in decision-making 55
common law 92
community, and sense of self 78
competence 11–12, 141
complexity, of decision-making 19, 211
confidentiality 98
Confucianism 18, 61–6, 67–8, 205
Confucius 61, 63–6, 67–8
consent 73–4, 124–31

Author Index